Remember Me

Living with Cancer:
A Story of Life,
Love, and Courage

Edward H. Cantor

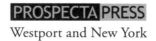
PROSPECTA PRESS

Westport and New York

First Edition

Hardcover ISBN: 978-1-63226-039-0

eBook ISBN: 978-1-63226-041-3

Prospecta Press

P.O. Box 3131

Westport, CT 06680

(203) 571-0781

www.prospectapress.com

Book and cover design by Barbara Aronica-Buck

Cover art based on image by Jasmina007

To Micki

and to Tom and Arthur, her warriors

Contents

Preface

Man Plans, God Laughs

On June 20, 2003, our life, as we knew it, changed forever. My wife, Micki, was a patient at Yale–New Haven Hospital undergoing surgery. The procedure lasted for more than four hours. The surgery involved several organs. The outcome was diagnosed as Stage III ovarian cancer. The cancer had spread beyond its original site.

It had begun with a simple ultrasound three months earlier. The results of that test were inconclusive. Ninety days later, after a second ultrasound, we were told that there was the possibility of a growth on one of Micki's ovaries. If the growth was malignant, the treating gynecologist advised us that she felt the cancer would be limited to one ovary. Several days later, surgery revealed the true picture—the cancer had spread to both ovaries and beyond. Our world was shattered.

Micki's life with cancer may have been similar to that of many other unfortunate patients who suffer from a lengthy terminal illness; however, for her, and for me, it was our only life. Her burden, over many years, was shared by her close family and friends. But it was the patient and me, her spouse, who were the main combatants in a long and torturous struggle with a deadly foe.

There were days of promise and rays of hope. There were standard procedures and innovative trials. It was clear that successful postsurgical treatment for one cancer patient would not guarantee success, in the future, for another patient with the same diagnosis, because cancer is an individual disease. After many, many years of research and of trial and error, we have learned that the fight against cancer will be won, one patient at a time. That dawn of a new era, the cure, would be too late for Micki. But I am convinced that the fight can be won.

Just as no two patients are alike, so are no two spouses, or partners, alike. What is a reasonable burden for one spouse may be unreasonable for another. And similarly, there is no one uniform way to grieve or mourn. Grief is a personal passage. It can be trivialized by those who are bystanders and who feel that they can prescribe the proper way to mourn the loss of a loved one. But they are merely bystanders.

In the beginning, in 2003, our world was peaceful and secure. My wife and I had been married for 31 years when our cancer journey began. We had one grown son and two grandchildren.

Micki had retired from her career in advertising at the

age of 57, some six years earlier. I had followed her in 1998 at the age of 58, concluding my professional life as the senior member of the Connecticut law firm I had founded. We felt financially secure, and we were ready to enter into another phase of our lives together.

Because I was a Yale graduate, both Micki and I were able to audit many courses at the university. We lived within 30 minutes of all university activities. The thought of exploring a whole new life was exciting, and, for the second time in our lives, we were transformed into college students.

Micki was attracted to courses in archaeology and ancient history. Those subjects had interested her greatly since childhood. She attacked the required and supplemental readings voraciously. She attended and participated in discussions with great enthusiasm. Her interest in and mastery of the subject matter were so obvious that a few of her professors suggested that she enroll in a degree program. Micki agreed, buoyed by their encouragement, and in 2001, she began the school year as a candidate for a master's degree in anthropology, with a focus on archaeology.

I was a less active student. I audited a course each semester, and did most of the reading, but did not write any papers or take any exams. I took a few initial courses in archaeology with Micki, but my interests were in a broader range of topics, from philosophy to history. A great deal of my time was taken serving on the governing boards of nonprofit organizations, none of which were related to my previous career as an attorney.

For a period of five idyllic years, Micki and I lived as students and volunteers. We vacationed from time to time. We tried to spend as much time as possible with our two young grandchildren, who lived nearby. We served as babysitters and drivers for them, read to them, and took them to destinations that young children enjoyed. We felt fortunate that they lived so close to us. One of the courses I took at Yale during this time was titled "Death." It was taught by Shelly Kagan, a brilliant young professor. I attended the lectures with about 300 undergraduate students. I had always been afraid of death and thought the course might help me overcome some of my fear. It did. In one of his final lectures, Professor Kagan told us that one of two things would happen at death: either there would be some type of a hereafter, or the person who died would pass into a state of nothingness. In either case, where there had been previous suffering, the suffering would cease. From that point forward, only those who survived would feel the loss.

I recalled that lecture many times after Micki's cancer diagnosis in 2003.

Man plans, God laughs is an old Yiddish proverb. Despite the best of plans, life does not always turn out as expected. We cannot control our fate.

In 1785, Robert Burns, the Scottish poet, wrote these much-quoted lines about the perils of planning:

> *But little mouse, you are not alone,*
> *In proving foresight may be vain:*
> *The best laid plans of mice and men*
> *Go often askew,*
> *And leave as nothing but grief and pain*
> *For promised joy!*
>
> (Standard English translation)

In 2003, our world was peaceful and secure. My wife and I were not prepared for the hostile and ferocious intruder that would force its way into our lives. That intruder was cancer.

This is the story of our trial with cancer. It is a story of hope and heartbreak. It is a story of love and courage. It is a story of failure and recovery. It is a human journey.

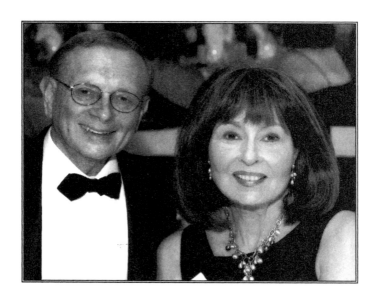

Chapter 1

Our Early Years

Micki was the older of two children, born to a middle-class Jewish family in West Hartford, Connecticut. Her father was a nuclear engineer. His career took the family from Connecticut to Oak Ridge, Tennessee, and to Schenectady, New York, during Micki's early teen years. She recalled that the moves left her feeling "rootless."

Her family structure contributed to a sense of insecurity. Her father spent little time with his children. His moods varied, and he had frequent fits of temper. From time to time, when Micki and her brother did not understand math or science as he did, he referred to them as "stupid." Her mother, Faye, through more subtle behavior, was equally destructive. Faye was a graduate of a college for teachers and clearly a bright woman, but she refused to enter the workforce and found the normal chores of cooking and cleaning to be beneath her. Neurotic and narcissistic, Faye absorbed her husband's verbal abuse by being passively aggressive. She usually won the private battles between husband and wife, and she took out her dysfunctional psychological tendencies on Micki and her brother, Richard.

For reasons that are difficult for me to understand, the chaotic family structure that destroyed a large part of Richard's life seemed to strengthen Micki's resolve. Micki and I talked about her childhood frequently. She had a clear understanding of the destructive nature of her parents' behavior and managed to survive and grow stronger.

At an early age, she exhibited strength of character. One episode that she recounted to me was illustrative. The family moved to Tennessee when Micki was about 12 years old. It was Bible Belt country. She was an isolated and attractive young Jewish girl. When she started her school year, she was approached by two young women who asked Micki if they could touch the top of her head. She asked them to explain their actions. They said that "all Jews had horns" and they were trying to find hers. Micki explained to them that Jews do not have horns—it was a myth—and that "we were all shaped by the same God." In recounting her story to me, Micki did not have any bitterness, but she had clearly been unnerved by the episode.

By the time the family moved to Schenectady, Micki was in the final few years of high school. She was tall, pretty, and bright. She had a flair for acting and was interested in the theater. She had a true stage presence, sang lyric soprano, and was endowed with perfect pitch.

As Micki approached college, she was hardly communicating with her mother and father. She had little in common with her brother. She recalled him as being reclusive. Her relationship with her father was obviously strained. Her mother presented her with a vexing dilemma. Micki felt a need to search for independence, despite a mother who was obviously manipulative and led her children to believe they were dependent upon her to make every major decision in their lives.

Micki spent most of her college career at Syracuse University. She was an acting and directing major. Her mentor, a noted dramatics professor, chose her for the leads in productions from Shakespeare to *The Mikado*—from dramas to musicals.

Later, when we talked about that time of her life, Micki said she felt that she was left with a personality that was torn by contradictions. She started with a family that did its utmost to undermine her personal growth. Her father berated her intelligence; her mother questioned her ability to make her own decisions. Her parents did their part in forming an insecure childhood, but her success in college did much to counter her insecurities. Her popularity and her physical attributes, combined with her successful acting career, bolstered her confidence. As long as she didn't return to her familial home, her growth and her career could flourish.

When she entered her senior year in college, Micki met and fell in love with a medical school graduate who was on his way to a residency in New Haven. They decided to marry as soon as Micki graduated from college. Their move to New Haven followed. About 14 months later, Micki gave birth to a baby boy, David. Micki was ready to postpone a promising theater career in the hopes of nurturing a happy and peaceful family. She desperately wanted something that she had missed in her childhood.

Shortly thereafter, however, her world caved in. During the pregnancy, her husband began to exhibit bizarre behavior. He changed his medical orientation from a career as a pediatrician to that of a pathologist—from a devotion to children to a career dealing with germs, toxicity, and death. He brought toxic substances home from the laboratory and insisted on keeping them in the refrigerator.

As Micki's pregnancy advanced, her husband's interest in his wife and future child waned. A few weeks after Micki gave birth and she and David returned home from the hospital, the break in her marriage was incontrovertible. David's biological father moved out of their apartment, leaving Micki and David to make it alone.

Several months later, the breach widened. David's father announced that he was leaving New Haven to continue his career in Tennessee. Micki was stunned to learn that he was more than willing to cut himself off from his wife and the child he had barely seen since his birth.

Micki was devastated. She was cut adrift emotionally and materially. Before her husband left New Haven, she was able to obtain a court order to receive the nominal sum of $28 per week for the support of David. Subsequently, she also received a small alimony order. Both awards were minimal. As a licensed physician, her now ex-husband was capable of making more money, but he chose to take a job in academia, which generated lower earnings. He argued, successfully, that he had less income available for alimony and support than a physician in private practice. Despite the small financial order that had been entered against him, as soon as he left Connecticut, he refused to pay most of the weekly amounts for alimony and support. Eventually, Micki was forced to go to Tennessee, where he was living, and hire a lawyer to collect the amounts that were owed to her.

I am at a loss to explain the behavior of such a despicable human being. I understand that many marriages do not survive. That is an accepted occurrence. But to emotionally abandon, in every sense of the word, a six-month-old child is beyond my comprehension. I know that David was a bright and engaging young boy. Even when his father was still in New Haven, in 1964, he rarely made any attempt to visit with David. His absence continued through the time that I married Micki in 1971. No visits, no inquiries, no attempts to sustain a relationship. It was not a human reaction.

David never knew his biological father. To a large extent, that was an unexpected benefit for me. There was no competition. David and I bonded quickly. I was, and I am, the only father that David ever knew. Our relationship remains close, loving, and proud.

• • •

The years between her separation and our first date were not kind to Micki. Her mother wanted her to return to Schenectady. Micki refused. She was determined to raise David on her own and knew that she could not return to live under the grip of her parents. They were able to provide very little financial support for their daughter and grandson, but from time to time they spent days with David. During these visits, Micki's father controlled his temper and her mother made a fuss over David.

After her first husband left Connecticut, Micki and David moved into a one-bedroom apartment. As David was no longer a baby, he occupied the bedroom while Micki slept on a sofa in the living room. There was very little income. Micki scraped together some money by singing lead soprano in a professional choir. She taught in a nursery school, and David was allowed to attend the school without cost. She began substitute teaching in public schools when David entered first grade. She dated occasionally. She had no emotional support and no family to rely upon.

Between the time that her brother, Richard, left law school and entered the Army, he was appearing less and less stable. He was living with his parents. David was about five years old when Micki's parents told her that Richard could no longer live with them and it was her responsibility to have Richard live with her and David. She succumbed to their pressure. Richard shared the bedroom with David and began to receive psychological therapy in New Haven. Micki found herself bringing up her young son while living with her brother's abnormal personality traits and unpredictable fits of anger. Fortunately, after several months, Richard left for the Army.

Micki and David survived those early years. It took great inner fortitude, and neither escaped the indelible toll that the period of years left on them. Micki was concerned with protecting David. She did not want him to be exposed to the lack of love and instability that she had experienced during her childhood. Remarkably, David, even as a young child, seemed to sense when his mother was being overprotective, and tried to strike a balance in their relationship. He was very verbal and challenged Micki when he found himself in an uncomfortable situation.

• • •

Micki and I met in New Haven in 1971. I was 31 and had never been married. I was a partner in a law office that I had founded, and I had few financial demands—I only needed to make enough money to provide for my expenses. I was very involved in the community. One of my nonlegal activities was as the campaign manager for a liberal Republican candidate who was running for mayor in New Haven. Micki volunteered to be a speechwriter for the campaign, which was how our paths first crossed.

It has often been said that opposites attract. From outward appearances, Micki and I were totally unalike. Micki was 5'9" in height. She made a stunning appearance. When she walked into a room full of strangers, she attracted immediate attention. She was substantially taller than I was. I often referred to myself as a "chubby little guy who lucked out."

Rabbi Mark Winer officiated at our wedding. Several years later, he was to write, "In a room of strangers, Micki and Ed would have been voted the most unforgettable. Physically, they were both extraordinary. Micki was every male fantasy of the ideal female, and quite tall. Ed, at under five feet, handsome and cherub-faced, was equally mesmerizing. Unforgettable, an impossible match, but irresistible! It was love at first sight, and in the epidemic of divorce convulsing the early '70s, few would have bet much on their marriage."

For Micki and me, it was indeed love at first sight. It was

a whirlwind romance: we met in August of 1971 and were married four months later. It was a union that, despite many odds, was to last for 39 years.

In many ways, one's parents become role models. In Micki's case, she was sensitive enough to realize that she needed to reject her parents as role models. My experience, growing up in Connecticut, was very different. Where her home life was tumultuous, mine was a sea of calm. My mother and father had great respect for and devotion to each other. I cannot remember one of them raising a voice to the other, or to my brother or me.

My father was very bright, but he did not achieve financial success or personal satisfaction in his work. He had graduated from college and law school in the middle of the Depression. He moved from New York to Waterbury, Connecticut, when he married my mother in 1935. His attempt to start a law practice ended in failure. Following that unsuccessful venture, he worked at several jobs that were not consistent with the educational level that he had attained, including driving a truck to deliver sand and gravel and working on an assembly line in a defense factory during World War II. Unhappily, he did what was needed in order to provide for his family.

My mother was an accomplished pianist as a teenager. She attended the Yale School of Music for a short time, but was forced to give up her formal education in order to take care of an ailing mother. After her marriage, she gave birth to my brother and, three years later, to me. From time to time she worked as a bookkeeper in a grocery store that was owned by her family.

In 1945, my father's parents opened a dry goods store in Derby, Connecticut, about 20 miles from our home. When my grandfather died a few years later, my father became involved in the store. In 1951, we moved from Waterbury to Derby. At that time, my mother also began to work in the business. Although my mother enjoyed her new job, my father found himself bored and unhappy. He was plagued by depression, indecision, and physical illness until he died in 1967.

Despite my father's depression and a lack of financial resources, even when both of my parents were working, I remember my childhood and teenage years as a series of happy events. My parents loved their children. Their primary goal was our higher education, and they sacrificed a great deal to that end.

When I reached the age of 12, we began to live in rented apartments. For a short time, we lived in a three-room apartment with my grandmother—five of us altogether. We rarely took vacations. We shared one car, and we were the last family on the street to acquire a television set. When my mother or my father had a birthday, instead of giving presents to each other, they made a contribution to the "education fund." At a time when many mothers stayed at home to raise their children, we were a two-person working family. But my parents always had time for my brother and me.

I was not aware of the despair over our financial concerns that my parents must have discussed behind the closed doors of their bedroom. It was never shared with my brother or me. I never felt deprived. I never felt poor. Feeling poor or feeling wealthy is a state of mind. It is all relative. We laughed together. We played together. We celebrated together. We were showered with love and affection.

Despite the ongoing financial difficulties, when my parents thought we should have music lessons, we had music lessons. When we needed to have our teeth straightened, they paid for it. Secondary school presented a challenge, however. They wanted both my brother and me to attend the best college that accepted us. Derby High School was not noted for its academic excellence or college preparation, so my parents sacrificed again and chose to send us to private schools for our secondary school education. My brother spent four years at Taft, a boarding school, and, three years after he started, I attended Hopkins, a private day school in New Haven. After Taft, my brother went to college at Yale and then on to Yale Medical School. I followed my schooling at Hopkins by spending my college days at Yale; I then went to law school at Columbia University. Some of our educational costs were covered through school loans and scholarships, but the rest were paid by my mother and father.

To this day, I am amazed that my parents could have accomplished so much with so little. I do know, because I eventually saw their tax returns, that my father never earned more than $9,000 in any given year.

In retrospect, my parents gave us much more than a good education. They gave us warmth and security. I grew up with the feeling that few goals were unattainable.

In that respect, I was very different from my father. Beset by personal depression and facing the economic Depression, he was not willing to take risks. He looked for stability and financial security. He had experienced a lifetime without either. In contrast, my parents gave me the confidence to make decisions and a willingness to take chances. I looked forward to being independent and shaping my own future. Attending Hopkins, Yale, and Columbia played no small part in creating that attitude.

When I graduated from law school, I was hired to work for an experienced attorney in New Haven. I was earning a respectable salary, but after one year I knew that I wanted to shape my own destiny. I did not want to have someone telling me what to do. At the time that I decided to open my own law office, my father was dying. I told him about my decision, thinking that I was sharing good news with him. To my surprise, he was visibly upset. He could not understand how I could forgo financial security (I had a good job) and risk the unknown. That episode illustrated a basic difference in our attitudes toward life.

• • •

I had been in my own law office for about five years when I met Micki. My outlook on life had not changed. Although our marriage did not conform to the accepted norm in many ways, neither of us was afraid to make the decision to marry.

David was then eight years old, and I saw him as an added bonus to my relationship with Micki. Yes, there were a few episodes of David "testing the boundaries" with me, but we quickly adjusted to life as a family. We sought to provide David with the love and security that was given to me as I was growing up but had been denied to Micki. A year after we were married, I adopted David. I was the first father that he really knew, and he was the son that I always wanted. Over the years, our close, warm, and loving relationship has flourished. For me, the best three-letter word in the English language is DAD.

The three of us built our life together. I was no longer the bachelor who could come and go as he pleased. Micki, David, and I were always together. I took pride in David's search for independence, and Micki gradually learned that she could not control his life. Micki and I disagreed, at times, over the degree of David's "striking out on his own." Those discussions always took place without David, and Micki and I were always able to reach an agreement. We tried to define boundaries and went through the same growing pains that were faced by most families.

When David left for college, Micki returned to work. She had substantial verbal skills and eventually held an executive position as the sales manager for a local cable television franchise. Under her leadership, the gross income generated by her division increased more than fourfold within a few years. Her tenure in cable television survived several changes in ownership and lasted until she retired in 1997.

At the age of 57, Micki had finished a successful career, had sent a son to college, and was looking forward to new horizons. She had found fulfillment in a life that was totally different from her childhood. It seemed as if the world was her oyster.

Chapter 2

The Diagnosis

Micki had entered menopause at a relatively early age. To counter the common symptoms of "hot flashes" and the bodily changes that often accompany menopause and continue for some time thereafter, Micki's gynecologist had placed her on hormone replacement therapy for several years. Around 1970, this therapy frequently consisted of the use of two drugs—Premarin and Provera. Premarin contained estrogen, which by itself could thicken the uterine lining. That buildup, or growth, could cause a proliferation of potentially malignant cells, so it was generally prescribed in conjunction with Provera, which could reduce the buildup.

In the case of Micki's cancer, her extended use of hormone replacement therapy was the first of a few specific "what-ifs" that occurred to me after her diagnosis. For many years, it was an accepted theory that hormone replacement therapy not only eased the "hot flashes" that occurred with the onset of menopause, but also was beneficial in reducing both bone loss and the risk of heart attack. Over time, these added benefits were questioned and even disputed. Furthermore, prolonged use of hormone replacement therapy was identified with an increased risk of breast cancer and a possible increased risk of ovarian cancer. Many practitioners felt that prolonged use of hormone replacement therapy could be harmful; they advised discontinuing it after a certain amount of time. Micki was advised of the risk; however, because of her extreme discomfort without the therapy, she chose to continue it. What if, I wondered, Micki had discontinued the use of hormone replacement therapy after a few years? Would her risk of ovarian cancer have been reduced?

For some time, while using hormone replacement drugs under the supervision of Dr. R., at the Yale Health Plan, Micki was given only estrogen through the use of the Premarin patch. Standard medical procedure would have called for the use of both Premarin and Provera (progesterone), but Dr. R. failed to prescribe the Provera. This deviation from typical practice continued for several months before it was discovered. Whether or not it could have accelerated the development of the cancer remains another unanswered question, another "what-if."

Ovarian cancer is notoriously deadly. Unfortunately, its early stages are frequently marked by no symptoms. Therefore, when the disease is finally detected, it has usually spread beyond its original site. Cancer is an uncontrollable growth of cells, and when the cells grow beyond their original location (metastasis), the disease becomes difficult and frequently impossible to control. The earlier that cancer is detected, the greater the chance of a cure or successful treatment.

In the late winter of 2003, Micki complained of some low back pain. She had always suffered from chronic back symptoms related to her discs and arthritis. She was referred by her gynecologist to Dr. Lynwood Hammers, a well-respected radiologist. Dr. Hammers administered an ultrasound test. It showed increased vascularization, an increased occurrence of blood vessels or blood flow, in the area of her ovaries. Dr. Hammers said that the condition was slight and that it should be watched for 90 days. Her gynecologist concurred. At the end of 90 days, it was too late. The cancer had metastasized.

What if Micki had simply undergone a hysterectomy at the time the ultrasound detected increased vascularization? If the cancer had been present then, would it have been contained to one ovary and not have metastasized? There would have been little risk in performing an earlier hysterectomy. At Micki's age, she did not need her ovaries. The options were not explained to us. We were never given the choice.

Ninety days passed. During that time, we told only our son about our concerns and did not share those concerns with others. After all, we had been told that nothing was conclusive.

We had been through a cancer scare before. About 20 years earlier, when Micki complained of back pain, an ultrasound had detected a potentially malignant cyst on the tip of her pancreas. She had surgery at that time, and the cyst was found to be benign. Knowing that nearly all cancers of the pancreas are fatal, we felt we had dodged a bullet.

Micki demonstrated her very strong character at the time of the pancreatic surgery. She gathered her close family together and told us, on the eve of surgery, that she was prepared to accept the findings, whatever they were. While I trembled outside of her presence, I kept up an optimistic façade when I was with her. She was courageous and maintained her dignity. She did not want to dwell on the possible diagnosis. Her main concern had been that her immediate family be looked after by our friends. In 2003, she faced surgery in the same brave and dignified way. Before her surgery, and during the course of her entire illness, I never heard her utter a word of self-pity or ask "why me?" Her courage was incredible.

In mid-June, another ultrasound was performed. We were told by Micki's gynecologist, Dr. R., that the results showed a nodule on the right ovary. She told us that it might be nothing, but, as a precaution, Micki should have an immediate hysterectomy. She assured us that the diagnostic test indicated that any tumor that was present was confined to the right ovary. I felt helpless, as if I were along for the ride. I had ceded control of our lives to the medical system and could only hope for the best.

• • •

June 20, 2003. I can't recall many worse days. Micki was scheduled to go to the hospital at 10:15 a.m. for surgery at 11:30 a.m. The hospital called us at 8:30 a.m. to confirm the schedule, and then again at 9:15 a.m. to ask where we were. Micki replied that we weren't due for another hour. The scheduler told us that we were wrong—we should have arrived at 8:30 a.m. It was not a good omen.

We left for the hospital immediately. Surgery started at 10:39 a.m. and continued until about 2:30 p.m. David joined me at the start of surgery to help me get through the suspense. We did not receive any news until about 3:00 p.m. At that time, Dr. R., the gynecologist, told us that cancer had been found on both ovaries and also on the omentum, a free fold of the peritoneum (the membrane lining the abdominal cavity) connecting the ovaries. Both ovaries and the omentum were removed, as well as Micki's fallopian tubes, which also contained traces of cancer. No other cancer was visible; however, the extent of the cancerous invasion could not be fully determined until all of the laboratory reports were in—a process that would take about five days. It was clear that the cancer had metastasized from one ovary to the other, as well as to the omentum and fallopian tubes. Dr. R. told us that Micki would need chemotherapy.

David, who had been fairly successful in keeping my mind on other things during the surgery, asked how the findings affected me. I had been somewhat optimistic going into the surgery based on conversations with Dr. R. I told David that I had accepted, in my mind, that there was a fifty-fifty chance of finding cancer, but the fact that cancer had been found on both ovaries and in other contiguous places came as a complete shock to me. It was contrary to what we had been led to believe. During Micki's pre-operative exam, Dr. R. told us that she thought the nodule that had appeared on the right ovary was encapsulated. We assumed that her statement was good news, considering the circumstances. Before surgery, we thought that if the nodule proved to be cancerous but was encapsulated, the cancer had not spread. Now, after surgery, we were being told that the tumor on the right ovary was no longer being described as "encapsulated." We appeared to be in a full-blown battle. I told David that I was more than concerned, I was devastated. Our faith in Dr. R., Micki's gynecologist, was substantially eroded. Several times, her version of medical findings was given to us with "rose-colored glasses."

I was faced with a situation that I had not experienced before. During our adult life, except for Micki's brief pancreatic scare, she and I had not been faced with a health crisis directly affecting either of us. Now we had to cope with a life-threatening disease, and the situation was made much more difficult by attempting to deal with a sluggish, insensitive medical bureaucracy. Over the years, physicians who were friends of mine had warned that we "would be better off if we were not in the system." Now, whether we liked it or not, we were being sucked into that ineffectual system.

I grew more frustrated as we waited for Micki to leave the recovery room. We were not allowed to visit her there. A volunteer was in charge of the telephone and help desk in the family waiting room. She was a sweet 80-year-old lady. Each time she called the recovery room to inquire about Micki's move to a private room on the surgical oncology floor, the traffic person in the recovery room told the volunteer that she was busy and would return the call. In the meantime, I was growing more and more impatient. I was concerned that Micki would be alone when she was told that she had been diagnosed with a metastasized cancer. After 30 minutes I asked for a supervisor, told her of the situation, and said I would file a complaint if I did not see my wife soon. The situation was resolved by the supervisor immediately, and Micki was taken to her room.

We had been advised by Dr. R. and others that a private duty nurse was not necessary during the first night after surgery. We were assured that the nursing staff on the oncological surgery floor was excellent. Although they were understaffed, it was true that most of the nurses on the floor were highly skilled. Nevertheless, we worried that any problems or unusual discomfort that arose during the night might not be addressed. A chair in the room opened into a small convertible bed, and I decided to stay overnight with Micki in case she needed help. I was concerned for her, and worried that she would be petrified if she awoke alone.

I decided that I, rather than any of her doctors, would be the one to tell Micki about the negative results of the surgery and the spread of the cancer. She was groggy after being moved from recovery to her own room, but she asked me immediately about the findings. I told her that cancer was found on both ovaries and the omentum and that all those organs had been removed. I also told her that there was no cancer visible to the naked eye elsewhere. It was a very difficult moment. We both knew that individual cancer cells were not visible and that if one had gotten loose, it was likely that cancer would eventually spread throughout her abdomen.

For Micki, that first night was uneventful. She slept most of the night. For me, it was sleepless and cold. In retrospect, I think that the chill I felt may have been caused by exhaustion, by a fear of the unknown, or simply by worry.

• • •

The next day was Saturday. We were told that a member of Micki's oncology team would visit her between 8:00 and 9:00 in the morning. No one appeared. At 9:30, I asked for an oncologist. He had been to the floor, had looked at Micki's chart and had left orders, but did not intend to see us. Dr. Tom Rutherford, her oncological surgeon, was not on call. In response to my request, the oncologist who was on call was located and came to the room, followed by a retinue of residents. He advised Micki that both ovaries were affected and that the course of treatment would depend entirely on the pathology reports.

It was then that I realized Micki had no recollection of my conversation with her the previous evening. She had been heavily sedated, and she still assumed that if there had been any cancer, it had been isolated to one ovary. She was devastated all over again once she realized that the cancer had spread.

The enormity of the situation struck both of us. Reality had set in. I was no longer merely "disappointed." We were both tearful and extremely depressed. Shortly after our discussion with the oncologist, our daughter-in-law, Abby, arrived to allow me to go home for a few hours. As I left the hospital, I realized that I was very angry and wanted to scream at someone. As I was driving, I was actually hoping that someone would get in my way.

On the way home, I dwelled on the loss I might be facing.

Micki's cancer could affect both of us in so many ways. I felt badly about the terrible physical and mental strain that was placed on Micki, but found that I was also worried for myself. A few days earlier I had thought that I could be strong and optimistic, regardless of the surgical results. Now those thoughts were shattered. I was falling apart like putty. Although the ride home only took about 25 minutes, it seemed as if a whole lifetime were passing before me. We had been married for 31 years. The love that we shared was, to some extent, taken for granted as we grew older together. Over time we spoke about it less frequently. Now, faced with tragedy, I realized how deeply that love was still alive.

A hot shower and change of clothes helped the strain. I returned a few phone calls from friends. It was difficult talking to them, and I could not get through a conversation without choking up. Nonetheless, their calls, messages, and offers of help were a great comfort. My support network was forming.

I returned to the hospital about three hours after I had left. Although a part of me wanted to stay at home and try to sleep for a few hours, a stronger urge was to be with Micki.

I was not prepared for the scene that greeted me in her hospital room. The previous evening, Micki had been taught to use the morphine self-medicating equipment to ease her pain. We were told that it was programmed to prevent an overdose and could be used every six minutes. While I was away, Micki had experienced a great deal of pain. She had been using the morphine pump at maximum frequency. She was extremely groggy, was not communicative, and could not open her eyes. She did not have the strength to draw water through a straw and into her mouth. It was clear that she had overdosed on the morphine accidentally. Utilizing the morphine pump at its maximum level, she had placed herself in a nearly unconscious state. The nurse was unaware of the problem and had not looked in on Micki for some time. The morphine cartridge had been emptied.

No immediate steps were taken by the nurses to remedy the situation. I spent the next two or three hours prodding Micki to stay awake while I hoped that the effects of the morphine would slowly dissipate.

Coincidentally, Micki was scheduled to walk for the first time that morning. We were told that she was to take three short walks on the floor during the day, but, after the morphine episode, she could hardly sit up without toppling over. By the middle of the afternoon, she had not walked at all. Fortunately, a doctor appeared and ordered an automatic drip of fluid to gradually remove the morphine from Micki's system. An hour later, we began to notice improvement. By 6:30 p.m., she took her first assisted walk and then collapsed in bed for a short nap.

Abby and David decided I needed a break that night, and I agreed. Abby stayed overnight. Thoroughly exhausted, I went home and slept for more than eight hours.

The first few days in the hospital revealed something that would be clear throughout Micki's illness: a sick patient needs a continual advocate. Sometimes the task could be as simple as holding her hand or getting her a drink. At other times, the need would be more acute—making sure that medication was administered on schedule, calling a nurse or aide when she was in pain and the staff was not responding to the call button, or coordinating a discharge to our home or another facility. I was able to attend to those details. I knew that, from time to time, it was necessary to make some waves in order to get the desired result. Frequently, I thought of the difficulty that would have confronted a sick patient without an advocate available. Plenty of patients become victims of the hospital bureaucracy because no one is present to support them or because they look on medical professionals as gods and are afraid to challenge them.

The nursing care was a problem, not because of a lack of quality care, but because there were far too few nurses and health aides available. At one time, the telephone at the front desk on the oncological surgery floor went unanswered for about 60 rings. No one was available to answer a call from a patient. We had superb nurses, but they simply had too many patients in need of care. I kept wondering what would happen if there was a true emergency.

• • •

On June 22, 2003, two days after Micki's surgery, I arrived at the hospital at about 9:30 in the morning. David and Abby were there. Micki was very alert and much stronger physically. We had been told again by all of her doctors that she needed to ambulate more, but inertia and depression had set in, making it difficult to get her out of bed. Still, we pushed her to walk because the nurses didn't have the time to do it. Eventually, we were successful in our efforts, and she took a short walk, trailed by one of us and her constant companion—her intravenous fluid on wheels.

Later that day, our cousin Ruth and our friend Eleanor came to visit. They were both cancer survivors, and their support was priceless. At one point, Eleanor looked around the room and said, "Except for Ed, all of us in the room are survivors." Micki answered her by saying, "I'm not a survivor." Ruth and Eleanor disagreed. To them, surviving the surgery meant you were a survivor. It was a state of mind. I don't think Micki ever looked on herself as a survivor. In the depths of her mind, as she said in later conversations, she felt that she would never be a survivor. When faced with looking forward to a good result or a poor result, Micki's outlook of a "glass half empty" usually prevailed.

That night, I ate a light supper by myself in the hospital cafeteria. When I returned to the 10th floor, I saw a face that looked familiar. It was my old friend and college classmate, Frank. He looked as if he had aged overnight. He told me that his wife, Mary, had been operated on for ovarian cancer two days before Micki. Her surgery had lasted several hours longer than Micki's, and Mary's problems were incredibly complex. I returned to Micki's room thinking that, as bleak as I perceived my problems to be, someone else's problem was always worse.

Cancer cases are rated in stages, according to their severity. Stage I might be a tiny, encapsulated tumor, with a great likelihood that the patient will survive. We were to find out in a few days that Micki's cancer had been categorized as a stage III cancer, giving her about a 50 percent chance of surviving for five years. In stage III cancer, cells have spread from the original site.

Mary, who had a very large tumor removed from her abdomen, was diagnosed as having a stage IV cancer. The odds, statistically, were heavily stacked against her surviving for more than five years. I had been at Mary and Frank's wedding more than 40 years earlier. As I write this, I am happy for my friends that Mary continues to survive. She is a testament to the fact that statistics cannot control your life. There is always the possibility that a patient will end up on the positive side of the equation.

Micki had a lot of pain that night, which did not subside until dawn. I stayed in Micki's room, but got very little sleep. I felt as if I were sleeping with one eye open.

• • •

By June 23, 2003 (three days after the surgery), I was convinced that if Micki stayed in bed for most of the day, her pain would take much longer to subside. At the risk of becoming totally obnoxious, I urged, cajoled, and insisted on getting her up to walk. I solicited the staff to make demands on her. It finally worked.

That interplay between us was a pattern that would be repeated many times during her illness. It reflected a basic difference in our outlook. She saw the glass as half empty; I saw it as half full. Her perception, as it applied to her own illness, may have been more realistic, but I refused to live my life that way. If the shoe were on the other foot, I hope that I would have responded with the same positive outlook, but no one really knows until his or her own life is on the line. One thing is clear—many people delay their physical recovery unless they have an advocate who is pushing them. The patient cannot always do things alone, and the hospital staff is usually too busy to do it for them.

At 10:00 a.m., the gynecologist, Dr. R., came to our room and confirmed that Micki would be moved to a step-down facility at the Yale Infirmary. Micki was well enough to leave the acute care hospital, but not well enough to go home. She still needed to have continual nursing care, wound care, and laboratory tests. I was very pleased with the move, knowing that the longer Micki was required to stay in the hospital, the greater the chance of infection. Dr. R. told us that Micki was a member of a very large club that no one wanted to join—a club of survivors. Dr. R. said that it was normal to cry or be depressed, and she encouraged us to seek the help of a therapist to help us adjust to our emotional needs.

As we were getting ready to leave, I had two other conversations. First, my friend Frank, who was arranging for his wife's transfer to a skilled nursing facility, told me that in all his planning, he had never imagined that he would survive his wife. I think that almost all my male friends shared that thought. Statistically, they were correct.

On an even sadder note, I was waiting in the corridor when I heard that a new patient was being admitted. I recognized the name: Shirley Barton. Shirley and her husband, Jack, lived in our town. We were friends, and we saw them a few times each year. I knew that Shirley had been fighting cancer for some time. Since we had not seen her for several months, we were unaware of her current situation. Jack came to Micki's room and told us that Shirley was being admitted to the hospital only because she was on her way to the Connecticut Hospice in Branford to die, but all the beds there were fully occupied. It was a very tearful encounter. Yet in all his sadness, and at one of the most difficult times in his life, Jack was caring and unselfish toward Micki, wishing her good luck in her recovery.

During our initial hospital stay, Tom Rutherford, the surgical oncologist, was difficult for me to find. He was the person who had "had his hands inside" Micki, and I was anxious to talk to him. I was frustrated by my inability to have a conversation with him, but did not want to risk alienating him, knowing that great demands were placed on his time and that he was the physician who would prescribe chemotherapy for Micki and continue to examine her at scheduled visits.

• • •

On June 24th, I went home to sleep, shortly after Micki was registered at the Yale Infirmary. I felt comfortable that she would receive a lot of nursing attention. School was not in session, and there were only three or four patients on the entire floor.

It was very strange for me to wake up in the middle of the night and not see Micki in bed next to me. We had been married for more than 31 years, and we had been separated for very few nights during that time.

I woke up early and planned to leave for the Yale Infirmary right away. But before I could leave the house, the telephone began to ring continuously. I heard from many friends, including some who had been out of touch for several years. The word of Micki's illness had been spreading quickly. I was particularly touched by a message from Paul Kennedy, the eminent Yale historian and scholar. During the last year, I had become involved with Paul's International Security Studies group. Paul had lost his wife to cancer a few years earlier. I had planned to meet him for lunch in a few days, but cancelled the meeting due to Micki's surgery. He expressed his concern and hopes for a good recovery and offered to "walk, talk, and kick a tree." I told him I would take him up on it.

While I was driving to the infirmary, I started breaking down emotionally. I had been running on adrenaline for a few days and had held many of my emotions in check, particularly in front of Micki. When I arrived at the infirmary, Micki was also crying. The events of the previous few days had caught up with her too. During her entire illness, it was one of the few times that she lost control of her emotions. We were scheduled to meet with Dr. Arthur Levy that day, and the following day Micki would be transported back to Yale–New Haven Hospital to have a port inserted. The port was to be surgically implanted under the skin. It was to be used during chemotherapy and blood tests, for access to the bloodstream, rather than having to locate a vein in the arm for each infusion or blood draw. It was a more direct way of receiving medication.

The oncology nurse, Molly, told us to expect six chemotherapy sessions, each three weeks apart, for an

18-week period. She told us that Micki would lose her hair. The fight had begun.

We had many visitors that day. As the day continued, Micki was noticeably cheered. She put on some cosmetics, changed out of her hospital nightshirt, took a shower, and gained strength. Initially, she had said that she did not want visitors; however, I recognized that she was much less depressed when people visited. Discreetly, I began to encourage people to visit her.

I had practiced law for more than 30 years in Connecticut, where most of the lawyers work in fairly small offices. In that situation, your ability to succeed is dependent on more than knowing the law. People often put their lives in your hands, and it is essential that you understand how to relate to them as you jointly make decisions that affect their lives. In law school, there is no course called "how to relate to people." Many lawyers have practices that do not flourish because they lack that very important human dimension. And so it is in medicine. I do not know of any medical school course given in "bedside manner." A doctor is entrusted with the most important thing a patient possesses—the patient's life. Frequently, the patient and his or her family are confused, shaken, and in need of reassurance. At the very least, the patient needs to know that her physician cares. I believe that the mental well-being of a patient and her family are second only to physical cure or improvement. A feeling of confidence in one's physician can certainly help in making a recovery.

Dr. Tom Rutherford was a superb surgeon. Over time, we came to know him as a trusted confidant and concerned caregiver. The longer Micki was his patient, the warmer the relationship between Tom and Micki and between Tom and me became. However, the very beginning of our relationship was a rocky road, largely due to the hospital bureaucracy.

Following Micki's surgery we were told, on several occasions, that Dr. Rutherford would be coming to talk to us. He never arrived. He was an elusive shadow. Later, I learned that he had seen Micki early in the morning on several days, but she did not remember the encounters. On the afternoon of the fifth day following surgery, we were told that Tom would telephone us within the next few hours with the results of the pathology tests. I was furious. As anxious as we were to learn about the results, I did not want to hear them on the telephone from a doctor we had never met. I spoke to the oncology nurse at the infirmary. She agreed that the telephone was not a good way to receive potentially heart-breaking news. The nurse spoke with the head of the Gynecology Department at the Yale Health Plan, Dr. David Roth. He agreed to speak with Dr. Rutherford to learn the results and then discuss these results with us. Dr. Roth came to Micki's room to tell us that he had spoken to Dr. Rutherford, but the results would not be available until the following day.

We were faced with another day of suspense and trepidation.

• • •

June 25th was a day of waiting. In the morning, Abby called to see if Micki was ready to visit with our grandchildren. At that time, Josh was nine and Zoe was seven. We delayed the visit. We did not want to see them until we had received the pathology report and had time to understand its significance. We also needed to figure out the best way to expose them to the fact of Micki's illness. They were young and had not yet faced the mortality of a very close relative. To Josh and Zoe, their grandmother was a warm, effusive personality. She had been attractive and vital before her surgery. How would they react to seeing their grandmother with tubes coming out of her, on oxygen from time to time, pale and weak? Whenever our grandchildren had seen her prior to surgery, Micki was bursting with energy. Now she could not stand or walk. She could not carry on lengthy conversations. It was an effort for her to stay awake.

Late in the afternoon, we were visited by Dr. R. She told us that the pathology tests confirmed the presence of cancer in both ovaries, the omentum, and the fallopian tubes. The good news was that the tests showed no spread of the cancer into the lymph nodes, and both the cervix and uterus showed no traces of cancer. Micki had a stage III cancer. It was strange to feel a sense of relief when you were told that cancer had been found at four sites, but we were relieved that there had been no lymph node involvement. Through reading and conversations with doctors I knew that the survival rate increased markedly if there were no traces of cancer in the lymph nodes.

Micki and I both knew that the chemotherapy would be very difficult and we had a long battle ahead, but there was some light at the end of the tunnel. Consistent with our differing outlooks on life, Micki said that fifty-fifty odds were very depressing. On the other hand, I pointed out to her that the statistics were only numbers. Fifty percent of the patients survived. Why couldn't she be one of the lucky ones? No one was able to give us the statistics for the survival of stage III ovarian cancer patients if they had been fortunate enough to survive for the first five years.

Chapter 3

The Treatment

On June 26, 2003, we were scheduled to meet with Dr. Arthur Levy, the oncologist who was to administer the chemotherapy. He would also examine Micki frequently. I had known Arthur for some time and was delighted that both he and Tom Rutherford would be monitoring Micki.

Although it had been several years since I had seen Arthur, he was as I had remembered him—a very caring person and a gifted clinician. He had an excellent bedside manner. He examined Micki and talked to her about the chemotherapy. He was very easy to relate to, but did not minimize the seriousness of the illness. He warned us that we were in for a long struggle and that the chemotherapy would have continual side effects. Arthur never lost sight of the fact that the emotional needs of the patient, and her family, were sometimes as important as tending to the patient's physical needs.

I told Arthur that I was confused by the conversations we had had about the possibility of curing the ovarian cancer as opposed to other talk about treating it as a chronic disease. He said that he had treated some people who seemed to be cured, but the more common result was to manage the disease for a long time. I did not want to ask him what he meant by "for a long time." He told us that the initial course of chemotherapy would last for several months, and it was important that Micki get through the first two years after surgery, when a high percentage of recurrences tended to occur.

Arthur told us that further surgery might be necessary to see if there had been any internal changes or if more cancer had appeared. That was not welcome news. We also knew that there would be continual monitoring by way of CT scans. Those diagnostic tests carried their own inherent risks by giving high doses of radiation to the body.

At the time, most ovarian cancer patients were tested for the presence of cancer by a blood test, referred to as the CA-125 test. A small percentage of patients do not register initially on the CA-125 scale. Unfortunately, Micki fell into that category. When she was given the CA-125 test shortly before her initial surgery, no markers were present.

Arthur said that he was cautiously optimistic. I was hoping for more optimism, but Molly Meyer, the oncology nurse, told us that Arthur tended to be conservative, and he never promised more than he could deliver. Nonetheless,

Micki and I liked him and Molly, and we knew that they would be very supportive emotionally.

Molly Meyer was a force of nature. She was a take-charge person. There was nothing that would stand in Molly's way as she sought to provide the best care for the cancer patient. She was a true professional, a teacher and a motivator. At a crucial time in their treatment, all the cancer patients at the Yale Infirmary came to know Molly as their advocate, protector, and friend. They would never be disappointed.

Micki's mother, Faye, was 84 years old at this time. She was totally alert mentally, totally neurotic, and totally narcissistic. She had suffered at least two heart attacks, had had bypass surgery, and was operating on about 25 percent of her heart capacity. Micki was her primary caregiver, and my mother-in-law and I did not have a particularly warm relationship. In order that she would not be alarmed, we had decided *not* to tell her about Micki's pending surgery. However, when we learned of Micki's cancer diagnosis and subsequent chemotherapy, we knew we had to tell her mother the bad news. We also decided that I was the logical person to do it.

I saw no sense in delaying our conversation. My mother-in-law was living in a senior assisted living facility. Before we spoke, I contacted the medical staff at the facility and prepared them in case Micki's mother reacted poorly to Micki's diagnosis. I was concerned about creating a medical emergency.

Fortunately, narcissism prevailed. My mother-in-law's reaction should have been predictable. She showed little concern for Micki and proceeded to tell me about her own illnesses and assure me that everything "would be all right"!

I called Micki on my cell phone to tell her that her mother was doing well. Micki told me that a nurse had just advised her that she was progressing to the point where she could be discharged from the infirmary by the end of the day and could come home. While waiting for all the paperwork to be completed, we were seen by a nurse and given home care instructions. Included among them were: "No heavy lifting, minimize climbing stairs, no driving, *nothing in the vagina*." That gave us a laugh! Sex was the farthest thing from our minds at that time.

• • •

It was good to have Micki at home again. That night, we both woke up at about 3:00 a.m. It was a tender moment, full of raw emotion. We reached for each other, ready to express our feelings. No topic was out of bounds for me, including my fear of her death, but Micki did not open up beyond admitting that she was aware she might not survive. I encouraged her then and many times later to talk about her fears with me, but she was reluctant to do so.

She usually maintained her dignity and control, even

when we were alone. She was not prone to hysteria, either before or during her illness. The closest she came to exhibiting sadness to me was frequent depression. For long periods of time, she became (understandably) quiet and withdrawn. The depression lifted when she was with our son and grandchildren and with friends.

In her relationships with friends, Micki decided to be very open about her illness; however, she did not want people to feel bad for her. She did not want people to treat her as "Micki, the cancer patient," but as "Micki, the person." She insisted people come to our home to visit and engage, but not to console her.

In retrospect, I think that Micki made up her mind, very early in her illness, to travel alone, to take her own journey from life to death. It was very clear that she wanted to fly solo. She was adamant about sparing her family, including me, the pain and anguish that she chose to internalize. Even in front of her husband and son, much less friends, she was determined not to break down. She refused to discuss her illness in detail with anyone. Maintaining her dignity was a way of controlling the situation, and a way of challenging death. She accepted that death waited in the future, but, as much as possible, it was to be on her terms. Till the time came, she was going to stare death down.

Unfortunately, that resolve did not make life easy for me. It was like having an 800-pound gorilla in the room and ignoring its existence. As I had that night we awoke together, I encouraged her to talk with me, but usually to no avail. I would have preferred her to unburden herself, but I did not want to cause her any more pain.

• • •

On June 27, a week after the surgery, we returned to the hospital to have the port inserted. It was to remain in place throughout chemotherapy, serving as an easy entry point to infuse chemicals or to draw blood. The alternative would have been to draw blood or inject chemicals intravenously. That method could wear out the veins or result in burning of the skin if some of the highly toxic chemicals escaped.

The port procedure went well. We then drove back to the Yale Infirmary where the oncology nurse removed Micki's stitches. Micki was doing remarkably well. The doctors advised total bed rest at home for the next three days, with minimal walking. We were both exhausted and had no problem with this medical directive.

The next day, David visited us at home with our two grandchildren. Our anxiety about our grandchildren seeing their grandmother in a debilitated state was for naught. They treated her exactly as she wanted them to—as if she hadn't changed at all. After talking to Micki, they swam in our pool and stayed for supper.

Before the surgery, I had exercised regularly. Since the surgery, due to all of my caregiving responsibilities, I had not been able to exercise for about 10 days. I took advantage of David's spending time with Micki and swam in the pool for 30 minutes. I also had intended to go to the final concert at the International Festival of Arts and Ideas that night, and Abby had planned to stay with Micki. As the day wore on, the people who were to attend the concert with me called to cancel. I was relieved that I was no longer obliged to go out that night. I really felt that I wanted to be with Micki. I knew that I would feel guilty if I was out while she was confined to bed. It was my first confrontation with guilt related to her illness. There would be many more in the future. In fact, much of my personal schedule and lack of activity would be controlled by feelings of guilt.

• • •

On June 29, I got up early and played two hours of tennis. It felt good to take out some of my pent-up aggression on the court. Micki stayed in bed all day. She was not very responsive to any attempts at conversation. Her answers were brief. She appeared to me to be depressed, but took several calls from friends.

I received two unexpected and emotional telephone calls. The first was from Phil Pivawer, whom I had known for many years. Phil was a first-class scientist, and I knew that his wife, Barbara, suffered from ovarian cancer and continued to decline. Phil had heard about Micki's diagnosis, and he offered his help. Tom Rutherford had been his wife's oncological surgeon and also administered chemotherapy to her.

Phil had done a lot of research about ovarian cancer. He educated me about several possible courses of chemotherapy and told me that he admired Tom Rutherford as a surgeon and clinician. When she was first diagnosed, Barbara's ovarian cancer had been much more advanced than Micki's. Barbara had exhibited symptoms and the cancer had spread to her lymph nodes and near her liver. She was now on her fifth different course of chemotherapy. She had never been in remission. Despite her torturous history, Barbara had just played 45 minutes of tennis. Phil and Barbara still held out hope that they might be able to continue to manage the disease as a chronic illness. Sadly, that was not to be; Barbara died a few months later.

The second call came from Joe Zelson, a local pediatrician. Micki and I had known Joe and his wife, Myra, for years, although we had not socialized with them for some time. Myra had been diagnosed a few months earlier with breast cancer. She and Micki were using the same oncology group. While most of my conversation with Phil that day had dealt with scientific and medical aspects of ovarian cancer, my discussion with Joe was more personal. He and I shared our respective episodes of waking up in the middle of the night to attempt to talk to our spouses and thinking that our marriages had not yet lasted long enough to end. Subsequent conversations with Phil were equally personal.

Both of these calls touched me greatly. Now, like our wives, these old friends and I had joined another club that no one wanted to belong to—we were spouses of cancer patients. Both Barbara and Myra had made the brave decision not to hide their illness. Micki had made the same decision; she would not hide the fact of the surgery or its outcome.

Later, I also spoke with my brother, Fred. He was a neurologist in Maryland and had two friends who were oncologists. I wanted to talk to him to get a realistic outlook about the coming treatment and possible outcomes. Arthur Levy, our oncologist, had said that he was "cautiously optimistic." What did that mean? Fred had offered to discuss Micki's pathology report with his colleagues, but he and they couldn't tell me much more than Arthur already had. The fact that Micki's cancer had metastasized was certainly bad news. Fred stressed that I should not dwell on the statistics. If 50 percent of the cancer victims survived for more than two years, Micki could fall on either side of that mark. On the other hand, that the cancer had not spread to the lymph nodes did not mean that some cancer cells were not floating around in Micki's system, waiting for the time when they could begin their deadly proliferation. It was hoped that the chemotherapy would be effective against any remaining cells.

After my initial discussions with doctors, Micki and I decided to look at surviving for the first two years after surgery as a realistic short-term goal. It was a topic that we had previously avoided. We saw the end of the first two years as a light at the end of a tunnel of gloom. If there was no recurrence during that time, it would be encouraging. Micki would endure two years of her own hell—chemotherapy, suffering the side effects, and the suspense of waiting for the results of periodic physical exams and CT scans. I didn't tell her that I would be suffering right along with her. She wanted me with her at every diagnostic test, every chemotherapy session, and every physical exam. There was no way that I could deny her that wish or my companionship. Micki had given me the gift of a life of 31 years of marriage. We were in this struggle together, as if we were joined at the hip. In my mind, that was what marriage was about.

• • •

By July 1, Micki's energy level was beginning to pick up. She had a CT scan to establish a baseline immediately after surgery so that doctors could compare subsequent CT scans to the first one to see if any changes had taken place.

Shirley Barton had died a few days after I had seen her

and her husband, Jack, in the hospital. That day, I attended her memorial service at a local church. As could have been expected, I wondered if this event were an omen of our future. Shirley had contributed much to her community. The minister said that the service was a celebration of her life, but it was difficult for me to think about celebrating.

• • •

That morning, we arrived at the infirmary for a 10:00 appointment, including a physical examination by the oncologist, to be followed by chemotherapy. Micki would be given Taxol and carboplatinum. The process was to take five hours. Micki tolerated the infusion very well. When we came home, I was totally spent emotionally. Each new procedure caused me to worry that a problem would occur. That pattern of thought had been established at the outset, when the initial surgery yielded results that were unpredicted and unwelcomed. In contrast, Micki had energy to burn. I could only guess as to its source: It could have been from the medication that she took to minimize the side effects of the chemotherapy, or it could have been an emotional reaction to having endured one round of poison. Temporarily, we had switched roles.

• • •

On July 4, Micki started the day feeling pretty well. She had been given steroids for pain, and antinausea drugs along with her chemotherapy. As the effects of the steroids wore off, she began to lose energy. She spent most of the day in bed. We returned to the Yale Infirmary at 6:00 p.m. for an injection of Neulasta—a drug that is intended to boost the production of white blood cells. White blood cells are essential to fight infection. Since the white blood cell count was usually low after every chemotherapy infusion, we were told not to go to the movies or any gathering of a large number of people. We could not put Micki in a situation where the risk of infection was increased. The retail price of Neulasta was about $2,000 per injection. Fortunately, because of the Yale Health Plan, we had to pay only $400 for the procedure. After the injection, on the way home, Micki asked for a milk shake and a muffin. That was all that she would eat for the entire day.

The next day, Micki was totally wiped out. She was feeling the side effects of both the chemotherapy and the Neulasta. She was nauseated, and had a metallic taste in her mouth and flu-like pains all over her body. These side effects were to be expected; however, expectations did not make the aftermath of chemotherapy any easier for the patient. Nor did it make it easier for me to watch. The cycle of nausea, flu-like symptoms, and loss of appetite would reappear with every subsequent round of chemotherapy.

Two days after the chemotherapy, Micki consumed just one slice of toast and some ginger ale during the entire day. Toward evening, her appetite seemed to be improving slightly, but she did not have the strength to get out of bed. I now understood why cancer patients become rail-thin; their appetite simply vanishes as the chemo commences.

• • •

On July 7, we woke up early. Micki told me that she admired the way that Jacqueline Kennedy had died, without sacrificing her dignity and before she had crumbled away to nothing. At the time, I did not realize that Micki was drawing from Jacqueline Kennedy Onassis as a role model. Dying with dignity became a mantra that she would follow until the very end. Micki was a very strong woman; she would not complain nor would she run away from the reality of death. At the time, I didn't know how to respond. I told Micki that we didn't know what Jacqueline's prognosis had been. It may not have been as good as her own. I told my wife that she had much to fight for—I needed her and so did our grandchildren.

A few knowledgeable people had told Micki that facing cancer was to be the fight of her life. I did not know whether those people were talking about the fight for survival from the disease or the fight to get through chemotherapy. It didn't matter. It all blended together in one desperate struggle. Micki assumed that the reference was to the chemotherapy, which was her immediate source of pain. The chemotherapy patients sometimes referred to each other as "sisters from hell."

Meanwhile, Micki and I were involved in our own little tug of war. I told her that she needed to begin walking on a regular basis. She resisted, telling me she experienced pain and dizziness when she walked and was too weak. I kept pushing her and told her that if she did not walk with regularity, her recovery would be slowed and her condition might worsen. I am sure that she viewed me as a nuisance. I thought my actions were necessary for her recovery, even though I might have pushed her to be angry with me from time to time.

• • •

By July 8, Micki was much more alert mentally but had no physical energy. She had trouble walking to and from the bathroom. When she ate, she either ended up being nauseated or having diarrhea. Eventually, various kinds of medication brought those symptoms under control.

We had an appointment with Micki's internist. Micki was so weak that I had to take her into the building in a wheelchair. We thought her weakness was the result of the chemotherapy, but we soon learned it stemmed from another issue. While we were with her internist, the laboratory checked her white blood cell count, which had recovered to a good level. When the internist examined her and asked her to stand up, Micki's blood pressure plummeted. This was a sign of dehydration. She was told that she needed to increase the amount of fluids that she consumed. It led to a vicious cycle, however: Micki, weak and frequently nauseated after chemo, couldn't eat or drink. The less she drank, the more dehydrated she would become. The internist told us to increase her fluid intake that night. If her energy level did not improve, we would need to return the next day for an infusion of salt, sugar, and fluids.

While we were at the doctor's office, Micki struck up a conversation with Pam, a patient whom Micki had met previously. Pam was finishing her chemotherapy that day, and all her tests indicated that she was in remission. Micki and Pam spoke of their common symptoms from the chemotherapy, including pain in the joints and bones, numbness in the extremities, and low-level nausea. In a strange and perhaps perverse way, it was comforting to know that the symptoms were common and most of them would pass. However, the numbness in Micki's fingertips never went away.

On the way home, I said to Micki, "We had a good day." Imagine the depths to which we had sunk! I was delighted that the symptoms that Micki was experiencing were indicative of dehydration. In the scheme of things, that was a mild and solvable problem. After a series of calamitous events, I was willing to settle for a mere bout of dehydration! That was the new normal.

• • •

On July 9, Micki's nausea and diarrhea continued. We drove to the infusion center at the Yale Infirmary, where she was given five hours of liquid nutrition. When we returned home, Micki ate lightly, and then her diarrhea began once more. The vicious cycle had started again.

We returned to the infusion center for more blood tests, all of which were satisfactory. Micki was still very fatigued, and she was given an infusion of saline solution, which had an immediate positive effect.

When we came home, Micki received a telephone call from Myrna Baskin, a kind and gracious person we had admired for years. Many years earlier, Myrna had had a non-malignant brain tumor that was successfully removed. I knew that she also had suffered from cancer a few years ago. We had seen her at events since her diagnosis, and I was always impressed by her incredibly positive outlook on life. Myrna had heard that Micki had ovarian cancer. She told Micki that she too had been diagnosed with ovarian cancer three years earlier and that she had experienced a full recovery. Myrna said that she thought she had cancer for a year before it was discovered, and it was diagnosed at a fairly advanced level.

Her call was like a message from God. It was invigorating.

Here was a very vital and accomplished woman who had survived the diagnosis, surgery, and postoperative treatment.
She urged Micki to call her at any time. For the first time
since surgery, Micki had spoken to an actual ovarian cancer
survivor. Micki said the call was the greatest gift she could
have received at that time.

Still, complications plagued Micki's recovery. Micki
knew that she would lose her hair as a result of the
chemotherapy, and we were planning to go to New York City
to shop for a wig. On July 11, as we got ready to leave, Micki
collapsed to the floor, unable to move due to pain in the area
of her right hip and groin. Micki had a long history of neck
and back pain and had medication to control that discomfort. After an initial consultation with the physiatrist who
treated the neck and back condition, she was able to relieve
some of her hip pain by increasing her medication and wearing a lidocaine patch over the area in question.

We postponed our trip and purchased the wig the following day. Micki chose shoulder-length hair, similar in color
to her own. To look in the mirror and see a full head of hair
seemed to revitalize her. When we returned home, Micki
noticed that her left leg was swollen and red. She removed
the lidocaine patch. I read the description of possible
contraindications and noticed that a small percentage of
patients reported a reaction of hives or erythema—swelling
and redness caused by dilation of the capillary veins. She also

had itching all over her body. She took a dose of antihistamine and, gradually, during the night, the swelling seemed to recede. At the same time, she began to break out in hives. For the next three days, Micki stayed in bed in order to ease the pain in her hip. She plied herself with antihistamines and topical cortisone for the hives.

Within a few days, Micki seemed to recover well from her hip pain and hives, but by this time her hair was coming out in clumps. Micki had suffered another blow to her femininity. For Micki, it was a psychological issue, and it took me some time to become sensitive to the problem. A few weeks earlier, she had lost her ovaries and her fallopian tubes. To me, survival was the issue. I told her that I thought she was the same person I had married. I believed it. She was alive, and the life we had built together could not be destroyed by the loss of hair or other physical changes. But to this proud, attractive woman, the loss of female organs and hair signaled a loss of identity and an inability to exercise control over her own body and life. Psychologically, the loss was devastating, Micki told me.

Although Micki's hip pain had abated for a few days, we returned to see Dr. Levy, so he could examine the hip. He found no cause for the pain. We were told that her blood counts were elevated and that it was a good sign. But what did that mean? If the chemotherapy was working, wasn't it logical that the blood counts would be lower? I was constantly examining each statement for clues about Micki's progress. I frequently wanted to raise questions, but did not want to do so in front of Micki in the event that the answer was more bad news.

That night, Micki said that she felt a small nodule in the area of her right groin. It was near the area of her earlier hip pain, but not in the exact same location. I tried to hide my concern. With my limited knowledge of biology, I thought I remembered that the groin was connected to the lymph system. Was this a sign that a tumor was now surfacing in the lymph glands?

As I think back to those early days of our cancer experience, I recall that every change in Micki's body was a source of concern. Clearly, I overreacted to many false alarms. That heightened sense of concern led to many sleepless nights and worry-filled days. One night, when Micki got up at 4:30 a.m. to take an antinausea drug, I woke up with her. She went back to sleep, but I could not and found myself crying next to her. I got up and went into another room so that I would not wake her or upset her. I tried to do some meditation to relax and eventually slept fitfully.

It was difficult to hide my concern from Micki, but I knew that she needed every ounce of strength she possessed to fight this enormous battle and did not need me to add to her burden. It was up to me to face my concerns alone or to find someone else with whom I could share them.

Frequently, that person was my brother, Fred. He had infinite patience with me. I knew I was fortunate to have a brother who was not only a superb neurologist, but also a person who wanted to help. He lived about 300 miles away, so most of our communication was by telephone or by email—usually when Micki wasn't in the room. I knew that talking about her condition in front of her could be upsetting. And although I relied on Fred and his colleagues for some medical advice regarding Micki's condition, he also served as an outlet for me to vent my emotions.

In other situations, I spoke to close friends. They were sympathetic but had not shared a similar experience. One exception was my friend Les Seligson. A few years earlier, Les had been diagnosed with multiple myeloma, a form of cancer that is often fatal. We had played tennis together, and I had tried to stay in touch with him during his treatment and long recovery. He had undergone a brutal course of chemotherapy and a stem cell procedure. I knew that, at times, the effects of his chemotherapy left him crawling on the floor. During at least four weeks of treatment, he had endured continuous, 24-hour daily infusions, with a bag of liquid toxins strapped to his waist and injected into his system through his port. I was aware of the many bouts of extreme nausea, weakness, and fatigue that he had overcome. I also knew that, although his pain had been great, he refused to succumb. Les had fought back gallantly, and now, some 10 years later, he was still a survivor. Les was a great model for Micki. He was in constant touch and raised our spirits. Of all my friends, and I'm fortunate that there were many, Les understood the emotional strain that we faced every day.

• • •

On July 18, Micki could still feel the nodule and called Arthur Levy at his office. We were experiencing one of those times of suspense and anxiety that we had heard about. Each new pain was suspected as a recurrence or spread. I went into the shower, and when I came out, Micki's complexion was ashen. Arthur had returned her call. Because he had examined Micki in the area of the nodule the day before and had felt nothing, he doubted that a new lump had formed overnight. He urged her not to dwell on it. Nevertheless, it was there, and she couldn't help but focus on it.

• • •

By July 20, Micki had been spending more and more time in bed. Finally, I decided that I needed to express my concerns about her inactivity. I tried to describe to her the cycle (one of many) that she was in: The more tired she was, the more she wanted to stay in bed; the more she stayed in bed, the more tired she became. Again, I assumed the roles of primary agitator and cheerleader. Micki understood what I was trying to do. At times, we butted heads, and the conflict created tension between us; however, she knew I was acting in her best interest. At times, her head wanted her to be more active, but her body would not cooperate.

• • •

On July 23, I took Micki to her hairdresser to have her wig shaped. Most of her hair had fallen out, and she decided to have the rest cut off. At the time of her initial diagnosis, when she had learned that she would lose her hair, she had brushed the thought aside as a minor nuisance. Now, added to all the other problems that she was enduring, it was a decimating and traumatic event. She found herself in tears. I told Micki that looks were superficial and had no meaning for me. To me, she had not changed. But to her, appearance reflected how one felt about oneself. For Micki, it was an unusually emotional reaction.

Chapter 4

The Chemotherapy

The next day, we arrived at the Yale Health Plan for another examination by Arthur Levy and another round of chemotherapy. He looked at Micki's right groin, where previous swelling had occurred, and remarked that there was "an asymmetry between the right and left groin areas." He ordered a CT scan for the following week. Those words were exactly the ones we did not want to hear. We spent the next several days fearing a spread of the cancer, even though Arthur told us that it would be very rare for ovarian cancer to spread beyond the abdominal area. Micki then had six hours of chemotherapy, which she tolerated fairly well. She was getting used to the infusions and slept during some of the session.

In the middle of the afternoon, while Micki was receiving her chemotherapy, I left to visit with Paul Kennedy, whose wife had died of pancreatic cancer several years earlier. We spent more than an hour together, sharing our thoughts, and both of us ended up crying. We had been friends before, but now we had a special bond.

• • •

On July 26, another cycle began. Micki felt nauseated all day. The nausea was barely controlled by medication. By evening, her bones began to ache. This was 24 hours after the injection of Neulasta, aimed at increasing Micki's white blood cells. If this cycle was similar to the previous one, her nausea would subside by the next day, but the bone pain would continue for another two days.

• • •

Two days later, on July 28, Micki was supposed to have the CT scan that had been scheduled by Dr. Levy. For the previous three days, she had been in bed as a result of the chemotherapy and had barely eaten. As we left for the scan, Micki was very concerned about the area of swelling in her groin. She had the CT scan after an anxious, hour-long wait.

That day, we received a very thoughtful telephone call from Steve Wolfson, the cardiologist who was treating my mother-in-law. I knew that his wife, Susan, had been battling cancer for some time, but I did not realize that she too had ovarian cancer. Steve talked to both Micki and me and was very comforting. Susan had suffered from an aggressive form of ovarian cancer and had been in treatment and on chemotherapy for more than three years. Steve was in a position to speak with cancer experts all over the country. One of the most reassuring things he told us was that his many conversations with cancer experts nationally led him to the conclusion that the medical care that was given to ovarian cancer patients at Yale was as good as any in the country.

• • •

On July 30, we had an appointment with Tom Rutherford, the gynecological oncologist who had operated on Micki. I had never met him. If Micki had seen him in the hospital, she had been too groggy or in too much pain to remember. As far as we knew, we had been scheduled for postsurgery visits but had never been able to meet.

We approached the visit with some trepidation, but were pleasantly surprised by Dr. Rutherford's very warm manner. We did not realize that he had the results of the CT scan and were delighted to hear that the swelling in Micki's leg was not a spread of her cancer. Apparently, it was a collection of fluid resulting from the disruption of her lymph system at the time of surgery. Dr. Rutherford felt the fluid was encased in a cyst and the cyst was pressing on the femoral nerve, causing pain. He said that the fluid would dissipate over time.

That diagnosis made the pain much more tolerable, but the pain was still there and was incapacitating. The medication that Micki was taking for pain was only partially successful in making her more comfortable. So far, the most effective prescription had been suggested by my brother—lying on tennis balls to relieve the pressure.

During the first several months of our encounter with cancer, we rarely talked about the disease itself or about Micki's current health. It was not necessary to talk about the monster that shared the room with us, because it totally engulfed our existence. We were driven by the chemotherapy schedule, the reactions to drugs, and the constant parade of diagnostic tests.

Try as we might to resist, our life was controlled by the chemotherapy sessions. There was no spontaneity to our existence. As each session occurred, the cumulative effect of the chemotherapy was stronger, and Micki became weaker.

• • •

On August 14, another round of chemotherapy began. Micki had been unable to walk, because the collection of fluid had not receded and continued to cause her pain. To counteract the pain, Micki took tramadol, a drug that reduced the pain but caused nausea and digestive problems. In addition, because she was unable to walk, Micki was restricted to bed. Bed rest caused increased weakness. Chemotherapy caused increased weakness. The whole process seemed like one big trap to render the patient immobile and depressed. Micki could not seem to break the cycle. However, she refused to break down emotionally. At a point when she was limited physically, she refused to complain. I was also trapped, but my predicament was emotional. I felt like I was in a continual downward spiral of helplessness. It was as if I had been thrust into the middle of a tornado, and could not get out.

During most of my adult life, I had sought to be in control. I volunteered for leadership positions. I welcomed the opportunity to make decisions. Now I found that I was helpless. I was an observer, unable to affect the outcome. I was a bump on a log.

It was obvious to me that when Micki walked, her pain was excruciating, so I no longer urged her to walk. We would eventually need to deal with the consequences of no physical activity, but we could not do so at the time because of the severity of the pain.

Micki's primary physicians were oncologists. Their concern was to obtain a successful outcome with a course of chemotherapy that would eliminate any remaining cancer cells. It seemed to us that they showed little concern for the cyst that had developed, rendering Micki unable to walk. Their focus was on the big picture. Anything else was a nuisance.

Micki was having fewer side effects from the chemotherapy because of the many drugs that were available to counter her nausea and some of her pain. Most of her adverse reactions came from the injection of Neulasta, which occurred 24 hours after the dose of chemotherapy. The Neulasta was successful in boosting her white blood cell count, but caused a great deal of pain. Each round of treatment seemed worse than the last, and, with each round, additional days were required for the pain to subside.

Following the third round of chemotherapy, we received the good news that Micki would not need to take the Neulasta after her sixth round of chemotherapy. Since the sixth round would be the last, there was no need to speed up the process of increasing her white blood cells. So, although there were three more rounds of chemotherapy, there would only be two more injections of the dreaded Neulasta. However small, any good news was a relief.

While Micki was having her next infusion, I met our friend Phil Pivawer for lunch. His wife, Barbara, had been in chemotherapy for 18 months, and the doctors had been unable to get her into remission. Phil looked totally drained. Clearly, he had been beaten down.

As a scientist, Phil spent a lot of time reading about the latest ovarian cancer research and gave me some material to read. I made a tactical mistake by bringing this information to Micki and reading it with her. The results of the research were so dismal that they led Micki to question if the pain that she was enduring was really worth it.

• • •

On September 4, Micki was ready for her fourth round of chemotherapy. Despite the side effects, she had been tolerating the chemotherapy well. We thought the cycle would repeat again, but learned to take nothing for granted and not to assume that any procedure would be tolerated without incident.

Micki was still enrolled as a student in the master's degree program at Yale. Because her surgery and chemotherapy had taken place during the summer, she had not missed any classes. Now the semester was beginning. If she had not been ill, Micki would have been taking her regular course load. In her current state, though, it was impossible for her to continue classes, particularly because she could not walk. It was a difficult decision, but Micki realized that she would need to take a leave of absence. Attending classes had been a significant part of her life, and Micki was disappointed. I was more concerned about her daily struggle with cancer and her inability to walk.

Meanwhile, the pain in Micki's right groin was becoming intolerable. One of the doctors stated a refrain that we would hear many times in the future: "It is very unusual; it only happens in a very small percentage of cases." It seemed as if Micki was destined to fall into that undesirable small percentage of complicated cases.

There was no consensus about how to treat the problem caused by the cyst, or lymphocele, pressing on Micki's femoral nerve. Dr. Levy said that a nerve block might do some good, but he wanted to wait until after the next CT scan, which was scheduled for September 19. My brother felt that the nerve block, which is carried out by inserting a needle at the origin of the nerve or at a point near the area of pressure and injecting that area with a local anesthetic, should be attempted immediately. Dr. R., the gynecologist, had no recommendation, but agreed that the situation was intolerable. She said that she would consult with Dr. Rutherford, who had not seen Micki for a month.

After one and a half hours of chemotherapy, Micki began to break out in a rash across her chest—an obvious allergic reaction. Again we were told that this reaction "only occurred in a small percentage of patients." The infusion was stopped; the rash receded immediately, and Micki was placed on steroids for an hour. This was the first time she had such a reaction. When the chemotherapy was resumed, the rash flared again.

The oncology nurse advised us to go home. Chemotherapy was terminated for the day. Micki was told to take five prednisone (steroid) pills at midnight and five additional pills at 6:00 a.m. the following day; the chemotherapy would then resume at noon. By premedicating, it was assumed that the steroids would prevent the allergic reaction from recurring.

I set the alarm for 11:45 and gave Micki the bottle of pills. That's when we discovered a problem: although Micki was scheduled to take 10 pills during the night, the pharmacy had only placed four in the bottle. We did not know whether it was a simple omission or if the pills were a multiple of the normal strength.

We called the Urgent Care Desk at the Yale Infirmary. Fortunately, a nurse was on duty who was familiar with Micki's chart. She was able to obtain 10 new pills, and I drove to New Haven late at night to get them. Even the act of filling a simple prescription could result in an error. The bureaucracy had struck again!

All in all, however, the fourth round of chemotherapy went well. Micki tolerated the medications necessary to minimize the nausea and lessen the pain from the Neulasta, which seemed to emanate from her bones; however, the deep and agonizing pain in her groin persisted and occurred more frequently. At times, the pain was even a problem when Micki was lying down.

Dr. Jerrold Kaplan, then Chief of Medicine at Gaylord Hospital, was a physiatrist who had successfully treated Micki for several years for back and neck pain. He was a good friend and a wonderful, caring physician. With Micki's cancer diagnosis, he had made himself available at all hours. Jerry conferred with my brother, and they increased the regimen of medication in order to suppress the pain, but nothing seemed to work.

• • •

On September 12, I took Micki to Gaylord Hospital to have a nerve block performed. Having the procedure was a decision that Micki and I made without the advice of the oncologists, although we made sure that they did not see any danger in it. Initially, her doctors thought that the difficult-to-reach iliohypogastric nerve was involved. Now, with the route of the pain more clearly defined, my brother and Jerry both thought it was the femoral nerve, which started at the spine and branched out along the inner and outer thigh. Jerry tried a nerve block in the outer thigh, which numbed that area but did not lessen pain along Micki's inner thigh. A nerve block along the inner thigh carried more risk because it was close to a major artery. Nevertheless, Jerry performed the second nerve block without a problem and with immediate relief. Jerry told Micki to rest in bed for a few more days to allow the numbing agents to take effect.

Unfortunately, the nerve blocks provided only temporary relief. The pain returned, as excruciating as ever. Jerry increased the oral medication, but the pain continued. By

September 17, Micki had taken such a high dose of medication that she began to hallucinate. She woke up several times in the night and asked me if I had hit her! She told me that she had imagined a strange man standing over her, about to strike her. The next day, she took less medication, and I took her for a blood test. When we returned home, Micki slept for 18 hours, suffering from the combination of continual pain and a lack of sleep.

That evening, I had planned to meet a friend, Vince Teti, who had come from New Jersey for a meeting, but I cancelled our dinner because Micki was not sufficiently alert to allow me to leave her home alone.

• • •

On September 19, I was able to meet Vince for breakfast. He had been a classmate of mine at Yale and is a very serious and compassionate person. He attained a great deal of success in the financial world, but has never forgotten his humble origins. I have always found it very easy to relate to him. I told him that Micki's illness was the most difficult situation that I had coped with in my entire life. Vince responded by asking a piercing question: Did I have a fear of Micki dying? Was it that thought that made it so difficult? I thought about my answer for a long time and finally responded that I was not afraid of Micki dying. I was afraid of what Micki had to go through to get to the point of death. It was the process of dying, not death itself, that was the torturous struggle. If the final destination was death, the road to be travelled was, I feared, a difficult and painful one.

Vince's question stayed with me for the next eight years. I thought about it frequently and always came to the same conclusion: I had accepted the inevitability of death. We were all going to die. In some sense, we were all already dying, some at a faster rate than others. How we died was the issue that Micki and I were facing, not whether or not death would overtake us. I was afraid of the suffering along the way, which is often the case when one faces a cancer death.

That afternoon, Micki had an appointment for a CT scan at Yale–New Haven Hospital. Arthur Levy had originally scheduled the test in order to take a closer look at the swelling near her groin; however, Micki had also felt a swelling and soreness in her abdomen. This was a new symptom, and one that she thought could be a recurrence of the cancer. The diagnostic test was expanded to include her abdomen.

We arrived at the hospital in plenty of time and used valet parking in front of the main entrance. I told the attendant that Micki needed a wheelchair. Yale-–New Haven Hospital is one of the largest hospitals in New England, yet it took the staff 20 minutes to find a wheelchair! Once again, the bureaucracy and inefficiency of a large institution added to our frustration.

The CT scan confirmed the continued problem with the cyst in Micki's groin, but did not indicate any further sign of cancer in her abdomen. This latest symptom proved to be a false alarm, but not before it took us on another precarious ride of high emotion and anxiety.

• • •

September 19 was the 36th anniversary of my father's death. It is Jewish tradition to attend a service at the synagogue and recite a prayer for the deceased each year. I went to the service in the evening alone. It was very emotional for me. Usually, Micki would have accompanied me. We were always supportive of each other in such highly personal situations, but this year, she could not come with me for both physical and emotional reasons. Physically, she could not walk. Emotionally, she wanted to avoid a portion of a service that was dedicated to those who had died.

I felt that I was alone, although several people at the service reached out to me and expressed their concern. I cried silently throughout the service, particularly when we said a prayer of healing for those who were sick and when we recited the mourner's prayer. Obviously, when we prayed for those who had died, I had more on my mind than my father; I did not know if the surgery and chemotherapy would eventually be successful. The premonition of death was our constant companion. When I was not in Micki's presence, the thought of a long, painful, debilitating illness culminating in death overwhelmed me.

The pain in Micki's thigh and groin continued. If she tried to walk any farther than 20 feet, the pain became excruciating and lasted for at least an hour. Ice seemed to provide some relief, but it worked very slowly. Each time we went to see a doctor or to have a medical test, I had to get a wheelchair for her.

Dr. Kaplan recommended a visit with an interventional radiologist to see about having a spinal block or to receive more information about draining the cyst. To our great disappointment, the radiologist did not recommend either procedure. Even if successful, he said, the block would be only a temporary solution (neither he nor we were in favor of putting a Band-Aid on the problem). He deferred to Dr. Rutherford about draining the cyst. We were very depressed and looked to Dr. Rutherford for a solution.

• • •

On September 24, the quest for relief was repeated with Dr. Rutherford. Promptly upon entering his office, Tom advised us that lymphoceles were not drained in this situation because they immediately filled up again. He also told us that he had once attempted to insert a permanent drain, and his patient had ended up with an infection that he fought for 18 months. Tom reiterated that the fluid from the lymphocele would be absorbed eventually, but it could still take six or seven months. He recommended lymph massage, intended to stimulate the lymph system and encourage drainage, as well as upper body physical therapy, because Micki had lost all of her muscle tone and had no stamina.

This was one of the few times that we disagreed with Tom. We knew that he was basing his opinion on his past experience, which had not been satisfactory. He was thinking conservatively and did not want to risk infection in someone in as weak a condition as Micki. In the long run, he was concerned that a serious infection could be a much more serious problem than the inability to walk for several months. Yet he was not the person living with the pain. It was Micki who was chained to the bed. Occasionally, she was able to walk to the bathroom or to a chair in our bedroom. I was her caretaker, making her meals and doing all that I could to make her comfortable.

We had become attached to Tom Rutherford and Arthur Levy as our warriors, the key people who would fight to save Micki's life. We were ready, reluctantly, to accept Tom's judgment even though it meant that we would be facing several more months of a greatly diminished quality of life. It was unthinkable to us, at that time, to seek a second opinion.

• • •

On September 25, it was time for the fifth chemotherapy session. Before each infusion, blood was drawn to check the levels of red and white blood cells, among other things. This time, Micki's red blood cell count was too low, and she needed to receive a supplement. Red blood cells carry oxygen, and their lack might have been the reason Micki was becoming breathless with very little exertion.

The infusion center at the Yale Infirmary had developed into a congenial group, and there were always two or three regulars whom Micki recognized. The majority of patients were women. The most tragic figure was a young, beautiful woman who worked at the Yale Medical School. She had been on chemotherapy for some time, and nothing was working. Outwardly, she maintained a bright and cheerful outlook. She died within a few months.

All the patients sat in a large circle so they could talk while receiving their infusions. On this day, they discussed the well-meaning but often offensive remarks of some well-wishers. All the patients sounded off on those friends who called and wanted to dwell on the illness or philosophize about the importance of a "positive attitude." The patients knew that a positive attitude might make them feel better, but numerous studies had indicated that a positive attitude had no effect on recovery. All the patients said that they wanted to be treated as people, not objects. They wanted to talk about normal, happy events, not whether or not the chemotherapy was working. None of the patients wanted to be preached to, particularly by those who could not understand their feelings and had never experienced the disease.

I understood that patients needed to be in control of their environment. These women were suffering enough—physically and mentally—without an intrusion on their space. In fact, on many occasions, I had found myself "running interference" for Micki so that I could tell visitors before they saw her that she did not want to talk about her illness. On the other hand, I felt that some of these patients were being too hard on visitors or callers, who at least had made the effort to express concern and reaffirm a friendship. They had not disappeared from the scene in the face of adversity, as several people had after Micki's diagnosis. When I met those same people during her illness or shortly after she died, they were very apologetic. The usual refrain was: "I wouldn't know what to say" or "I didn't want to intrude on her privacy." I was not sympathetic to them. I knew all the excuses, because, at one time in my life, I had used the very same lines when friends were ill or hospitalized. I had stopped making excuses when I realized that my own fears or selfishness had made me afraid to visit those who had been stricken.

The "regulars" at the chemotherapy sessions also talked about food. They all said that their loss of taste varied from day to day. In general, they all experienced a loss of appetite. Micki agreed. She had some cravings, and I would try to satisfy them. However, if I brought in food that she craved a day after she requested it, she had often lost her appetite for it. One day, she had longed for cheesecake during chemotherapy. The next day I bought a cheesecake and defrosted it for two hours. When it was ready, Micki asked for soup.

This was a pattern that occurred frequently during Micki's illness. If the cheesecake episode had occurred while she was well, I would not have been very patient. However, I was involved in her battle with cancer as much as a spouse could be. I had committed to making her as comfortable as possible as soon as the cancer had been diagnosed. We were at another stage in our lives, and many of the earlier ground rules that had governed our relationship as husband and wife were thrown out the window. What might have resulted in a disagreement before Micki's illness was now simply a trivial nuisance. Patience became a byword, and we were able to laugh at those incidents.

• • •

October 3 was the bottom. Micki could not walk. She had not fully recovered from her last round of chemotherapy. She was on multiple drugs and was completely depressed. She was not communicative and was confined to bed. My friend Les called her. Because he was a multiple myeloma survivor and had completed six months of chemotherapy, Les and Micki had established a relationship. Where I had felt hopeless, at times, about connecting with her emotions, Les was able to speak to her about a shared experience. Although I was sympathetic, I had not experienced Micki's suffering. I was there to hold her hand when she was nauseated, to give her medication when she was in pain, and to clean up after a bout of vomiting, but I was going through a different kind of suffering—that of a loving but helpless onlooker. Les had been there. I had not. He had stared down death, and Micki was looking it in the eye. I was not. When she finished talking to Les, Micki hung up the phone and burst into tears. She had been controlling her emotions for weeks and broke down. All I could do was to hold her tightly.

On the same day, I had scheduled lunch with a good friend, a psychologist. Alan Lovins had been very supportive of me since Micki's diagnosis, and I found it helpful to talk to him. Despite Micki's highly emotional state, she and I agreed that I should keep my appointment. I felt guilty for leaving her alone, but I could not have anticipated her fragile emotional state when I made the date with Alan. It was one of the few times, during her entire illness, that Micki's stoic attitude abandoned her.

Yet later that afternoon, Micki's mood changed. She found that she could get out of bed for short periods of time without experiencing terrible pain. On the day that she had hit rock bottom, it appeared that she was beginning to claw her way back. Over the next few days, her outlook seemed to brighten.

Micki and I developed a plan of action. There were a few decisions that I felt had to be made by Micki. I could lay out the alternatives, but she needed to make the final decisions. It was her body and her life. I could work on the details and be supportive, but she had to participate.

One of those decisions related to getting a second opinion on her treatment. A college classmate, Bruce Chabner, was the clinical director of the cancer center at Massachusetts General Hospital, one of the best hospitals in the country. Bruce had earned an excellent reputation among oncologists for his cancer work at the National Institutes of Health and at Mass General. I had emailed Bruce a few weeks earlier about a protocol that involved injecting drugs directly into the abdomen following the initial course of chemotherapy. The idea would be to increase the patient's chance of survival by aggressively going after any stray cancer cells that were not killed by the initial series of chemotherapy treatments, I hardly knew Bruce, but as classmates at Yale we shared a common bond. Here was another situation in which I felt that a certain amount of good fortune eased our plight. He responded immediately to my emails and offered to have us come to see his colleague, Dr. Michael Seiden, who specialized in ovarian cancer research at Mass General. I had delayed responding to Bruce's offer until Micki was well enough to go to Boston with me. Having finished most of her chemotherapy at Yale, we felt that the time was ripe. She was in favor of considering a trial to improve her chances of survival.

On October 6, Mike Seiden called to discuss including Micki in a trial. Her involvement would commence as soon as she finished her initial chemotherapy in New Haven. Mike was very pleasant and thoughtful on the telephone. We scheduled an appointment with him and the chief of surgery for women's services at Massachusetts General.

• • •

We approached the sixth chemotherapy session on October 15 and 16 knowing that it was the last scheduled session in the initial protocol. All the people at the infusion center, patients and staff alike, knew that it was a milestone. Because Micki continued not to register on the CA-125 test to detect the presence of cancer, it was difficult to determine her progress, although all physical examinations had been satisfactory.

From time to time, some of the patients brought in food to share in a spirit of camaraderie. Since this was our last session, we wanted to do something for everyone. At first, we were inclined to order a cake, and we considered the inscription "the end" or "hooray." We decided that neither would be appropriate. "The end" could have more than one meaning. Superstitiously, it could be a curse. "Hooray" might be insensitive to other patients, who were now friends, who might never be able to celebrate because they had suffered a recurrence or had a poor prognosis. We opted for a big "6" to mark the sixth round of chemotherapy. Some of Micki's fellow students and faculty from the Archaeology Department joined us. They brought flowers and balloons. The event was orchestrated by Micki's favorite professor.

The infusion itself was not without problems. For the second time, Micki began to have an allergic reaction during the process. The infusion was interrupted, but Arthur Levy wanted Micki to absorb the full dose of chemicals. She was given steroids and an antihistamine and was able to finish her treatment.

Since the aftermath of the fifth chemotherapy session had passed with few problems, we hoped that the sixth would have a similar result. It did not. Micki had a great deal of leg and body pain.

• • •

On October 18, two days after the final infusion, we should have been celebrating. Micki had finished her course of chemotherapy. None of the treatments had been delayed or reduced. Arthur Levy was impressed, since he had given Micki the maximum possible dosage. Strangely, we were both left with an empty feeling. A friend asked, "What do you do next?" I said that we would pray. We had an initial two-year crucial period facing us. Although it seemed much longer, we had only made it through four months of the two-year period after diagnosis, when most ovarian cancer recurrences occur. While we were in the middle of the chemotherapy, we knew we were doing the most we could to combat our evil adversary. Now that we had finished the protocol, we felt helpless—all we could do was wait. Considering cancer trials for further treatment allowed us to be proactive and seemed like it might relieve some of our anxiety.

• • •

On October 27, we drove to Boston to discuss alternative treatment, including the possibility of becoming part of a trial. Micki was very weak, as expected. We had been told that she would probably experience weakness after the last blast of chemotherapy because the effects of the chemotherapy were cumulative.

Bruce Chabner had arranged for us to meet with Dr. Arlan Fuller, the Chief of Gynecological Oncology at Massachusetts General, and Mike Seiden, the head of clinical trials, who had spoken with us a few days earlier on the telephone. Bruce was also kind enough to join us. We were accompanied by our daughter-in-law, Abby. The doctors were patient and polite and talked to us for about three hours.

That day was my birthday. Instead of celebrating, we received some devastating news: according to the doctors at Massachusetts General, the cure rate for Stage III ovarian cancer was 35 to 40 percent. That was a more dismal statistic than the one that we had heard in the past. The definition of a cure rate was that the patient survived for five years after the surgery; statistics beyond five years of survival generally weren't available. Furthermore, they advised us that if a recurrence happened, the cancer would eventually kill the patient. After hearing that depressing outlook, I was numb, but did not want Micki to see my reaction. After all, I was the one who had continually reminded Micki that she could be one of the survivors in the wider group of all cancer patients. I was the one with the glass half full, but the facts that now confronted us left little room for optimism. To break the tension, and change the subject, Abby began to ask some relevant questions.

The doctors at Massachusetts General were conducting

a trial that was winding down. They told us that Micki could be included in it. This trial involved inserting ovarian cancer antibodies directly into the abdomen. The antibodies carried a radioactive ingredient and were intended to attach to and kill or neutralize any stray cancer cells. It was an interesting theory that had been successful in treating some blood cancers.

There were a number of problems to be considered. First, if we wanted to take part in the trial, we needed to respond quickly because the study required that the process occur within eight weeks of completing the initial chemotherapy program. Second, we needed to understand that it was a trial and the final results would not be known for another four to 10 months. Finally, and most importantly, there were significant potential side effects. A number of trial participants had developed bowel obstructions, and almost 75 percent of the cancer patients involved in the trial had suffered some permanent loss of bone marrow, which compromised the immune system. That could mean if Micki needed further chemotherapy because of a recurrence, her ability to tolerate the chemotherapy at a high level would be compromised. In such a case, should Micki enlist in the trial, it was possible that she might actually be shortening her life. Before deciding whether or not to participate in the trial, we wanted to discuss the procedure with our doctors in New Haven.

There was some hopeful news. Dr. Fuller examined Micki and confirmed that her groin and leg pain was caused by a large lymphocele pressing on a nerve, rendering her unable to walk. He wanted to drain it. We had been hoping for weeks that a doctor would attempt that procedure. We made an appointment to have the surgery performed, in a two-day procedure, a week later.

• • •

On October 28, we returned home and saw Tom Rutherford, who had previously refused to drain the lymphocele. Surprisingly, he had changed his mind, and he suggested that we have the procedure performed at Mass General. We asked him for his opinion on the proposed trial. He said that he did not believe in the antibody theory. He recommended doing nothing further at that time, since Micki had successfully completed the standard protocol for ovarian cancer without a significant adverse reaction.

I talked to Tom privately about the ovarian cancer survival rates that had been quoted at Massachusetts General. Although he did not deny the statistics, he said that Micki was at the high end of the spectrum. All Stage III cancers were included in the statistics, and that included patients with abdominal wall or lymph node invasion. Micki had neither of those problems. As far as Tom could tell, all the organs affected by the cancer had been removed. Nevertheless, we all knew that ovarian cancer was very aggressive. A few stray cells could have been resistant to chemotherapy. Those cells could eventually lead to uncontrollable cell growth and be life-threatening.

Memorial Sloan Kettering Hospital in New York City was running another trial, which involved an injection of chemotherapy directly into the abdomen once per month for four to six months. (Micki had received chemotherapy through a port under her collarbone.) It also had potential side effects, including possible damage to the kidneys. Tom was not in favor of the Sloan course of chemotherapy, either, but said that if we were going to choose between the two trials, he would pick the Sloan version.

We were thoroughly confused and concerned about the potential side effects of any other treatment. All chemotherapy involves the injection of toxic substances into the body. When you are dealing with toxic substances, there is no free ride. We felt like it was all a roll of the dice.

We asked Arthur Levy for advice. Unlike Tom Rutherford, he did not specialize in ovarian cancer and, for that reason, did not want to opine as to the potential benefit of entering into a trial. He did express concern, however, about any trial that carried a significant risk of damage to other organs or would weaken a patient's immune system.

Micki and I weighed the conflicting options. It would

have been easier for us if all the doctors had been in accord.

• • •

At the end of October, Micki's blood was tested, and it was clear that the chemotherapy had taken its toll. Micki's red blood cell count had plummeted. We were to return the next day for a blood transfusion. Within a day, her red blood cells had risen to a satisfactory level, in time for the lymphocele procedure that was planned at Massachusetts General Hospital.

On November 1, we returned to Massachusetts General Hospital. It was not one of my favorite places. In fact, it carried some very painful memories for me. In 1966, my father, age 59, had suffered from a neurological problem that resulted in a gradual deterioration of many of his bodily systems over a number of years. Fluid was collecting on his brain, prohibiting him from walking or controlling his bladder, among numerous other related conditions. It was determined that he needed to have a shunt inserted near his brain to drain fluid away from that organ and into his circulatory system. Mass General was chosen because it was close to our home in Connecticut and was one of the best hospitals in the country. In addition, my brother was a resident there at the time and would be able to watch over my father.

Prior to my father's surgery, a radiological procedure had

caused air to collect near his brain, and he was unable to speak. Acute glaucoma also occurred within several hours, and he lost his eyesight permanently. He was transferred from the operating and recovery rooms and was attended to by a private duty nurse. One day, his attending nurse took a coffee break, and my father, who was agitated, tried to get out of his bed. He fell and suffered bleeding inside his skull that increased the pressure on his brain. The shunt disconnected, and he fell into a permanent unresponsive state and remained in that condition, in the hospital or a nursing home, for about a year until he finally died. This was an agonizing recollection.

My second experience with this hospital occurred in 1984 when my son was attending summer school at Tufts University in Medford, Massachusetts. At about 2:00 a.m. one night, we received one of those telephone calls that all parents dread. A voice at the other end of the line said, "This is the Emergency Room at Massachusetts General Hospital. Your son has been in a motorcycle accident. He is in critical condition."

We left immediately for Boston and spent the next 10 days at David's bedside. He had bought a motorcycle without telling us and had been hit by a passing vehicle. He was thrown 60 feet in the air, landing on his head. Fortunately, he was wearing a helmet, which saved his life. He suffered some temporary brain trauma, a badly cut leg, and broken bones in his feet. Except for some loss of taste, he emerged, after several weeks, without a disability. The event was traumatic to us all, though the care at Mass General was superb.

There may have been some superstition involved, but those two experiences had left me unsettled. As we arrived in Boston for Micki's procedure, I was worried about several potential problems: the surgery might reveal a spread of the cancer, infection could occur, or her bowel might be punctured, since it was located next to the lymphocele.

Despite all my concerns, the initial procedure went well. The drain was inserted, and Micki spent the night in a hospital room. The next day, an attempt was made to collapse the lymphocele. If it was collapsed, it could not fill up again with fluid. Alcohol was injected through the catheter into the lymphocele. The intent was to irritate the lining of the lymphocele to the point that it collapsed. The results of that process would not be known for several days. The drain was left in place for days, allowing any additional fluid to escape.

We were sent home and scheduled to return in a week. After several days had passed, the volume of fluid being emitted from the lymphocele had not abated. We thought that the procedure had not worked and worried that it might need to be repeated—this possibility had been mentioned. If, after a second attempt, the procedure was still not successful, there were also alternatives.

Meanwhile, for the first few days, we were not sure that

the leg pain had subsided. Micki's blood levels continued to fluctuate, and she did not have enough strength to test her ability to walk. Before the procedure, pain occurred after about a five-minute walk and then recurred each time Micki attempted to walk for more than a minute. Until she had the energy for a five-minute walk, we could not determine whether or not the surgical procedure had been successful.

• • •

On November 6, a few days after surgery, Micki was strong enough to test her leg. She walked, pain-free, for five minutes. It was the first time in several months that she had been able to walk without crippling pain. We were overjoyed.

• • •

On November 10, the day before we were scheduled to return to Mass General, Micki began to spike a fever. Her temperature went up three degrees within four hours. I was very concerned about infection. Chemotherapy lowers the white blood cell count and weakens the immune system. Micki was easy prey for an infection, so we decided to leave for Boston immediately.

It was after 5:00 p.m., and most of the hospital departments were closed. Fortunately, my friend Bruce had given me his cell phone number. He answered after the first ring. He was concerned about the availability of beds at the hospital. Bruce told us to continue to Boston and assured us that someone from the hospital would call back within an hour. About 50 minutes later, we received a call advising us that Micki would be admitted and that a bed was available. We were indebted to Bruce for all his efforts on our behalf. Micki was admitted with a low grade fever and put on antibiotics.

• • •

The next morning, November 11, Micki required a CT scan before further work on the lymphocele. She was allergic to the dye used in CT scans and required steroids at six-hour intervals beginning 13 hours before each scan. That protocol was started during the night before the scan, which was scheduled for 10:30 a.m. The nurse who was on duty called the interventional radiology department to confirm the appointment and advise the diagnostic radiology office that Micki had been admitted to the hospital the night before. Unfortunately, that registration changed Micki's status from outpatient to inpatient. It would seem that this change should have been handled by simple paperwork, with very little effect on the patient. For a huge monolith like a hospital, however, there is no simple change. For a reason that seemed unfathomable to us, the change in status meant that she would be seen by an interventional radiologist later in the day. We pleaded to stick to the original schedule because of Micki's premedication requirements. We asked, continually, if the change in schedule would have an effect on the steroids that she had taken, and we were assured that there would be no change. However, when Micki was moved to the interventional radiology department at 2:30 p.m., she was told that she would need to begin taking steroids all over again. To our great frustration, we were moved from department to department. Micki was given steroids and antihistamines intravenously.

We felt that we were caught in "the system." During Micki's treatment, we were plagued by the web of bureaucracy. For a normal person, the frustration is nearly intolerable. For a patient who has been weakened by chemotherapy, exhausted by its side effects, and is facing life-and-death decisions, the frustration is inhumane. We felt abused.

I tried to be tactful. We were in the hands of doctors and technicians and did not want to alienate them; on the other hand, I told them that the administrative problems were placing an unfair burden on the patient. In a way, the scene was ironic. We had received superb treatment up to that point. But even the good name of my classmate, Bruce Chabner, could not overcome the bureaucracy that exists in nearly all hospitals.

When the interventional radiologist finally tested to see if the lymphocele had hardened and collapsed (a process called sclerosing), we were told that it had been only 50 percent effective. There was a chance that the lymphocele would fill up with fluid again, so the procedure was repeated later in the afternoon.

In the interventional radiology department, the physicians paid very little attention to the well-being of the patient after the procedure was completed. Micki was wheeled out to a corridor and waited for at least 30 minutes before someone arrived to take her to her next destination. That attitude was, to our experience, peculiar to that department. At every other point in our stay at Mass General, the level of care and concern was excellent.

We drove home that evening, feeling battered and beaten. When Micki and I talked, I tried to keep her in a positive mood. As had been the case with all her treatment since her initial diagnosis, she did not complain. I was not nearly as patient and forgiving, but I kept those thoughts to myself. I reminded Micki that we had achieved some measurable success. She was now able to walk.

• • •

Until November 14, Micki was in considerable pain. I took that as an indication that the sclerosing was occurring. I was scheduled to go to a luncheon and meeting in New York, but as Micki's pain persisted, it seemed less likely that

I would leave her. Fortunately, that morning the pain diminished. I went to New York but called Micki several times during the day. I felt guilty that I had left her alone.

• • •

On November 18, we returned to Mass General. We were under the impression that a test would be conducted to determine if the procedure had been completely effective. We were met by a new physician, Dr. James Wise. Much to our surprise, he did not perform another test. He simply removed the draining tube and told us that we were finished. When I asked him how he knew that sclerosing had occurred, he responded that he felt the process was complete based upon the pain symptoms we had described and the fact that the drainage had virtually stopped. Micki was eager to start exercising, but her doctors cautioned her against it. They told her to limit her exercise to walking for several weeks in order to allow scar tissue to form.

We returned home that night greatly relieved. We were indebted to Bruce Chabner, whose care and concern were a testimony to old college ties. He had paved the way for a surgical procedure that was not as simple as we had imagined. In retrospect, it was easier for me to understand the reason for Tom Rutherford's urging us to have the surgery performed at Mass General, which, by the sheer volume of its patients, had undoubtedly performed the procedure many times more than Yale–New Haven.

• • •

On November 19, we received an envelope in the mail from Massachusetts General Hospital confirming our appointment a day earlier! The directions in the envelope described the procedure as "tube injection," implying that a reverse flow would be injected into the drain to be sure that sclerosis had occurred. It was not my imagination. Now there was something new to worry about. Dr. Wise had chosen not to perform the tube injection. Instead, he had simply removed the tube based upon his own conclusions. I decided not to say anything to Micki about my concerns and threw the envelope and notice away.

Ultimately, Micki decided not to participate in either of the trials. We decided to cast our lot with the doctors at Yale, who had gotten us through the chemotherapy and with whom we were familiar. We were wary of any trial that could compromise Micki's immune system or affect a vital organ, knowing that the chemotherapy had undoubtedly taken its own toll. Later, we would learn that the trials at both Mass General and Sloan Kettering had not produced any conclusive findings.

Chapter 5

The Aftermath

The course of chemotherapy took less than five months, but seemed like an eternity. There would be no need for further treatment unless there was a recurrence.

Micki was able to walk again, without pain. She was very weak from many months of chemotherapy, confinement to bed, and lack of exercise. The chemotherapy had left her with very little hair on her head; it came back gradually, but she would never again have the pleasure of looking in the mirror and seeing a full head of hair. The light hair that had grown on her arms prior to the cancer would never return. She had lost some of her sense of taste and had a constant ringing in her ears that never went away.

In addition, Micki had a condition called lymphedema, marked by swelling of the legs. When she had her initial surgery, the doctors tried to determine whether or not the cancer had invaded the lymph glands. In the course of surgery, the lymph system was disrupted in her legs. This proved to be a permanent condition. If unattended, the affected leg can look like an "elephant leg." The condition is not uncommon among women who have had surgery for breast cancer, but in that case, an arm would swell.

None of Micki's doctors had warned us about the possibility of this condition, and, as it developed, they were slow to recognize it and offered little advice as to treatment. Understandably, they were concerned with the cancer. That was the killer. No one was going to die from lymphedema. However, the lymphedema affected Micki's quality of life; it was unsightly, prone to infection, and a constant reminder that one of her bodily systems was not functioning properly.

To cope with the swelling, Micki would wrap her leg in several elastic bandages to constrict the swelling. The bandages caused her legs to become overheated and uncomfortable and had to be changed daily. In addition, she would see a physical therapist trained to massage the legs, stimulating the lymph system and moving the buildup toward the kidneys and lungs, to be absorbed and expelled.

Wrapping and unwrapping her legs at the beginning and end of each day became a daily ritual for Micki. Psychologically, it was a constant reminder that she was not whole. I never heard her complain, except to mention her lingering feeling that her days as a "complete female" had passed her by. At no time did that loss of her own sense of femininity detract from my affection for her. I tried not to miss an opportunity to tell her so.

For the rest of her life, Micki continued to mourn the loss of her femininity. During one of our intimate conversations, she told me that she felt as if her womanhood had been ripped away from her. She had lost her ovaries. Her hair had fallen out and would never return to its original fullness. The lymphedema left her, from time to time, with heavily bandaged or swollen legs. Her body bore the scars of surgery. In my eyes, she was still beautiful, and I told her so. For an attractive woman who prided herself on how she presented herself, however, my words were of little solace.

Chapter 6

The Interlude

Micki was alive! We looked for a return of some degree of normality in our lives.

The medical system had controlled our lives, and we had felt that we had little independence or autonomy. From the day of the initial diagnosis to the end of chemotherapy, our lives had been tightly guided by a schedule set for us by medical practitioners. Suddenly, we were told that we could plan to live our own lives again.

The fight had become *our* fight. The treatment schedule was *our* schedule. The outlook was *our* outlook. Micki and I were in it together. When Micki finished her first course of chemotherapy, we had been married for more than 32 years. Our relationship was one of mutual love and devotion. There was never a thought that Micki would be left alone to struggle for her life. I would be with her. This was our shared burden. Our lives were more and more intertwined. I had terminated most of my voluntary activities during her treatment. Micki had been unable to continue her studies. I had felt thankful that I was retired and was not bound to a job that would have caused me to spend more time away from Micki.

When the chemotherapy ended, the mental adjustment was not easy. We had become dependent on others telling us where to be and what to do. While in the grip of chemotherapy, our lives were simplified. We knew that we could expect a day for the infusion, a few days of calm, several days of Micki's feeling wretched and confined to bed, a week to rebuild her strength, and then the cycle would begin all over again. While our routine was set for us, we had felt secure that there was nothing more for us to do. Once free of that obligation, we felt a sense of insecurity. Should we be pursuing further treatment? Had all the cancer cells been killed? Was Micki better off with the poison of chemotherapy coursing through her veins? We felt as if we were living in a sea of uncertainty.

Now, with chemotherapy concluded, we were left to pick up the pieces. Our medical obligations, for the foreseeable future, consisted of monthly physical examinations and periodic CT scans. Micki had to regain her strength and deal with wrapping her leg daily as a result of the lymphedema. She looked forward to the day when she could begin to exercise.

Freedom from the rigors of chemotherapy should have

been a cause for rejoicing. A few months after the end of chemotherapy, Micki was told that she should have her port removed. I thought it was a step along the way to recovery. To Micki, however, the port had become a talisman. As long as the port was a part of her, she felt, superstitiously, that it could ward off evil. Arthur Levy, one of Micki's oncologists, explained to us that any foreign body that was inserted under the skin brought with it the chance of infection. There was no choice but to have it removed, and Micki reluctantly agreed.

The months passed. Following my "glass half full" theory, I expressed enthusiasm to Micki with every passing month. It marked more time distant from the dreaded cancer. Following the "glass half empty" theory, Micki was certain that the cancer was lurking around the corner. She believed that we had not seen the last of the disease. Privately (although I never said it to her), I too felt that we were not rid of the plague. Because Micki's cancer had already metastasized at the time of its discovery, I felt that the chances of eradicating each and every cancer cell were small. Still, we talked about living our daily lives as if the cancer were gone.

Micki regained her strength slowly. Before the surgery, she had been a vibrant person, frequently seeking new areas of interest. When she was well, she was active in mind and body. She exercised daily for an hour at a time. Her body did not have an ounce of excess weight. She didn't smoke and rarely drank. She had an inquiring mind and read constantly. It was not unusual for her to read an entire book in a day. She was a student of ancient history, current politics, and, most of all, archaeology. She was eager to resume that life and move on from being the "sick person." By September 2004, she had resumed her classes at Yale. It seemed that as each month passed by, a tiny piece of the dark cloud lifted. Micki enjoyed interacting with young students, and several came to our home for dinner. Micki also had an excellent relationship with some of the faculty members, especially Frank Hole and Tom Tartaron. They were not only teachers but also became close friends and confidants.

Micki's area of expertise was the Levant, that great swath of land including parts of Iran, Iraq, Syria, Lebanon, and Israel. She was most interested in ancient cultures—about 6,000 B.C.E. Her thesis described two ancient societies, one succeeding the other. By analyzing fragments of pottery from both cultures, she sought to determine whether the succession had occurred by friendly integration or by a more intrusive method, such as war.

As a student of archaeology, Micki initially expected to spend time at an excavation site in the Middle East. In one of her early years of study, Tom Tartaron taught her the technique of archaeological excavation at a local dig in Guilford, Connecticut, but she was prevented from going to most of the Levant by the volatile political situations that plagued those countries. Yet, many digs were available to her in Israel, which we had visited several times. During one of our visits, Micki had been introduced to several prominent archaeologists, who had invited her to participate at their sites.

Almost all the digs in Israel operated during the summer months when the desert was dry and very hot. As a result, Micki's lymphedema prevented her from participating because of the danger of increased swelling and infection. It was a great disappointment to her, and, because of her physical limitations, Micki became a bench archaeologist. She grew skilled at identifying a small pottery sherd and matching it to a culture. I was amazed by her ability to take a small piece of the neck of a broken jug and draw the entire vessel.

As her stamina increased, Micki completed her coursework at Yale and moved on to her thesis. Much of her writing could be done on her own schedule, so we were able to do some traveling, and we took several trips within the United States.

Before Micki's diagnosis, we had visited Botswana with two very close friends, Nancy and Frosty Smith, and we had expected to return to Africa. In 2006, Micki and I decided to go to Tanzania. The trip was difficult for Micki. It set the limits of her endurance. We had gotten into the habit of taking an extra piece of luggage to hold the several sets of clean bandages that were necessary for Micki to avoid infection. We could not rely on the possibility of properly washing and drying bandages while on safari. Changes in pressure on the airplane to Tanzania caused substantial swelling even before we landed. Then, the weather was very hot and humid. To our dismay, both of Micki's legs swelled significantly. Micki spent days lying down, hoping the swelling would recede, unable to go out and see the wildlife.

It is difficult to go through the trauma of Stage III cancer and not be scarred. For the remainder of the time that Micki seemed to be cancer-free, we could not drive away the rain cloud over our heads. It lifted slightly at times, but it was always there. Although I kept my thoughts to myself, I was always waiting for the other shoe to drop.

Micki's preoccupation with the return of her cancer was ongoing, and I urged her to share her concerns with me. Rarely was she willing to be open. Though we felt close to one another, Micki still seemed to feel that her struggle with cancer was one she needed to face alone. Later, after her recurrence, she told me that she always had felt uncertainty about her chances of being cured. Yet she didn't need to tell me: I could see that she couldn't shake the air of sadness that was frequently with her when the two of us were alone.

There was a noticeable difference when we were visited by David, and by our grandchildren, Joshua and Zoe. Micki brightened every time they were with us. When Micki was first diagnosed with cancer, Joshua was nine years old and Zoe was seven. Micki worried that if she were to die within a few years, her grandchildren would be too young to form a lasting bond with her. She was concerned that they would never remember her.

Fortunately, that was not the case. Our grandchildren visited Micki when she was in the hospital at the time of her first surgery. They crawled into bed with her when she was feeling the effects of the chemotherapy. They were at our home regularly during Micki's remission, and they were with Micki until the very end. Gradually, Joshua and Zoe accepted Micki's illness as a part of life. It was a tribute to their parents that the children did not fear illness. All the love that Micki gave to them was reflected in their great affection for her. In the last years of her life, Micki knew that her concerns had been unfounded.

Though Abby and David divorced shortly after Micki's initial surgery, both agreed on the importance of their children's relationship with us. Micki was even able to preserve her relationship with Abby, who visited frequently.

As with me, Micki did not let down her guard in front of David. As our only child, he visited with his mother frequently. It gave me the opportunity to have some time to myself, and I urged them to talk together when they were alone. I know that David encouraged Micki to discuss her concerns, but she kept her thoughts to herself. It may have been a mother's protective instinct—to shield her child from unpleasant thoughts. She was as a shepherd, protecting her flock.

• • •

In February 2008, we were able to achieve a long-promised goal—a trip to Israel with our grandchildren. Joshua had celebrated his Bar Mitzvah in 2007, and Zoe was due to celebrate her Bat Mitzvah in 2009. As soon as our grandchildren had started their religious school education, we had promised them that we would go to Israel together. Micki and I had visited Israel several times and had even lived there for a few months in 1989. Neither of us could be considered religious, but the influence of our heritage and our fascination with the history of the country acted as a magnet that pulled us back.

From time to time, Micki needed a day of rest during the visit. On this trip, unlike the trip to Africa, that was easy to accomplish since we were setting our own itinerary and daily travel schedule. As a result, the trip was not physically exhausting, and we were free to enjoy the emotional and memorable experience.

Chapter 7

On Borrowed Time

In 1938, a play by Paul Osborn about the role of death in life was performed on Broadway. The play enjoyed several Broadway revivals and, in 1939, it was made into a movie starring Sir Cedric Hardwicke and Lionel Barrymore.

The play was set in a small town in America. Pud, a young boy, is left to take care of his elderly grandparents after Pud's parents are killed in an automobile accident. Death, personified by Mr. Brink, visits Gramps (Pud's grandfather) to put an end to the old man's life. Gramps resists Death, and lures Mr. Brink up into an old apple tree. Gramps holds domain over the tree and anyone who climbs on it. Mr. Brink is caught in the tree. He cannot leave without Gramps's permission. As long as Death (Mr. Brink) remains in the tree, no one can die. Gramps, although ailing and infirm, can continue to live.

The townspeople are skeptical of Gramps, but when several people who should have died manage to survive, even the town doctor becomes convinced of Gramps's power over

Death. The doctor points out that a world without Death will mean added suffering for those with incurable diseases, and for the infirm and the ailing; however, Gramps is unwilling to release Death.

Then, Pud falls from the fence Gramps has built around the tree and is paralyzed. Seeing the suffering of the young and the old, Gramps relents. He releases Mr. Brink from his tree. Death frees Pud and Gramps from a life of suffering and takes them to the far beyond.

The name of the play (and the movie) is *On Borrowed Time*. The main characters (Pud and Gramps) are living on borrowed time. Their lives are filled with pain. When Death is released, suffering and torment cease. Death becomes part of life—its natural conclusion.

I became aware of the play when I was 12 years old. By coincidence, it was experiencing a revival on Broadway in 1991 when my mother died. I took Micki, David, and Abby to see it because of the meaning it held for me.

When Micki was stricken by cancer, and as she suffered a long, slow slide toward death, I thought about the play many times. I don't know if Micki was on borrowed time after her initial surgery in 2003, but I do think she was on borrowed time after she entered into remission. Clearly, she was on borrowed time after she suffered her recurrence in 2009.

In a sense, we are all on borrowed time. It remains for each of us to make the best of it.

Chapter 8

Recurrence

In the summer of 2008, we were invited to a friend's
house for a picnic and were introduced to an oncologist
who had recently lost his wife to breast cancer. During
the conversation, we told him that Micki had been without
a recurrence for more than five years and that her doctor had
considered her to be cured. He responded tactlessly: "The
only way you know that you have been cured of ovarian cancer is when you die from something else."

Despite that reminder, we were gaining optimism at the
end of 2008. Micki had survived for five-and-a-half years
after surgery and chemotherapy. She had received positive
medical reports. Physical exams, CT scans, and blood tests
were becoming intermittent. Micki was progressing toward
her master's degree and was finishing work on her thesis.

• • •

On January 12, 2009, the struggle began anew. Micki felt a lump near her ribs on her right side. Our calendar had called for her to see Tom Rutherford at a regularly scheduled appointment in two days, on January 14. As Tom examined Micki, he could not hide his concern. Of all of his patients with ovarian cancer who had survived for five years, he told us, only one had suffered a recurrence.

Micki was destined to become the second. Tom ordered an immediate CT scan, which showed a mass next to her liver and, confusingly, not in the area of the rib where Micki had felt the lump. He ordered a biopsy. That procedure had some risk because the mass was located near her aorta and lung. The biopsy was negative, but Tom did not believe it. The size of the mass was alarming. In addition to the mass near Micki's lung, he detected a tumor near her upper intestine—the lump that Micki had felt near her rib. Tom was sure that the tumors were a recurrence of the initial ovarian cancer. He wanted to remove both of them surgically as quickly as possible.

I saw our good friends Frosty and Nancy that night. As soon as Nancy saw me, she knew that something was wrong. Nancy had become adept at reading my feelings. Though Micki and I had decided that we would not hide her illness, there were very few friends with whom we shared the details and our ultimate concerns. Nancy and Frosty were on that short list. They sensed when we needed them, yet were careful never to intrude on our privacy. It did not take me long to explain the new findings, and, as expected, they shared my disappointment. It was a comfort to be with good friends who had been there for us since the original diagnosis.

Surgery was scheduled for February 10. The delay was caused by the need to coordinate the schedules of the two surgeons, who would work simultaneously to remove the two tumors. Tom would remove the growth near the upper intestine. Dr. Ronald Salem, a liver specialist, would remove the tumor next to the liver. Micki was convinced that, once she was opened up, her doctors would find cancer all over her abdomen.

We did not go out of our way to tell people about the coming surgery. We called David on the way home from the doctor's visit and shared the bad news with him. We left it to him to tell the rest of our immediate family. David immediately told Katie, a woman he had been dating since shortly after his divorce. Katie and Micki had become close. He also told Abby. Micki's former and future daughters-in-law were both intimately involved in her care and were of immense help and support to me.

Whether by design or good fortune, I was building a tight network of family and good friends who would become irreplaceable as we faced a troubling future. Alan and Lynn Cadan were part of that group. Alan and I had grown up together in a small industrial town near New Haven. We went to grammar and secondary school together and were reunited when the Cadans retired and moved back to our area. Micki and Lynn had become fast friends. And then there was Sarah Lane, Micki's oldest friend, who lived in Florida. She and Micki had become close friends when Micki and I were first married. Sarah and her husband, Rod, were married at our house. During Micki's initial diagnosis and treatment, Sarah was a constant presence. Sarah referred to Micki as her sister. They laughed and cried together. Every week, during the last 18 months of Micki's life, she received a card or long telephone call from Sarah. Each month during Micki's last six months, Sarah flew from Florida to Connecticut to visit her.

If I had to draw a diagram of my male friendships, I would probably draw concentric circles, each filled with several names. My closest friends were part of the innermost circle. Micki's circles would have been fewer and smaller. She tended to draw a small group of friends to her, but, if you were part of that group, she would move heaven and earth for you.

We turned to our closest groups of friends as Micki faced the beginning of the end. The night before her surgery, we planned a simple dinner with Nancy and Frosty. When we finished eating, they asked Micki if there was anything they could do for her. "Yes," she answered, without wavering, "I don't know how this surgery will turn out. Just take care of Ed."

Micki was beyond being concerned about herself. My wife was the bravest person I had ever known.

Micki remained incredibly stoic in the face of surgery. She knew that the outlook was dismal. The findings of the surgery would predict whether she had weeks, months, or longer to live. But the ultimate result was never in doubt. She was truly on borrowed time. A few days before the surgery, Micki and I discussed the future. She said that she did not want to look too far down the road. She told me that she was prepared to die, but that she still had a few things she considered unfinished business, including Zoe's Bat Mitzvah, scheduled in about four months, and completing her degree.

It was during that conversation that Micki again set the tone for her outlook on her remaining days. She did not want to talk about her health. She wanted to talk about life—what was happening around her.

Micki also wanted to put everything in order. She wanted to have little things in the house improved for me so that I would have no problems living in the house or selling it in the future. On the eve of her surgery, Micki insisted on writing letters to me, to David and our grandchildren, and to our niece, Claire, whom we loved as if she were a grandchild. Micki insisted that the letters not be opened until after her death. I put them aside and honored her wishes. She seemed in control of her future. From that point on, she rarely talked about her health. She asked me to make it clear to visitors that health was not a subject to be discussed.

Appearance was very important to her. She wanted to appear as Micki, the living person, rather than Micki, a woman on her way to death. In fact, after she died, her friends told me that their conversations with Micki never touched on her illness or eventual death.

• • •

The surgery on February 10 took more than six hours. To reach the tumor near the liver, Dr. Salem had to cut Micki's diaphragm and stitch it back together. David stayed with me in the family waiting room. Tom Rutherford came out of the operating room to see us after four hours; he was optimistic. He said that, to the eye, the tumors appeared to be encapsulated and both had been removed intact. As far as he could see, Micki was "cancer free," although, of course, he could not determine the presence of any microscopic cancer cells. He was relying on his visual examination only.

Tom told me that the cancer had not infiltrated Micki's bowel or liver. Although he had not mentioned this before the surgery, he had been concerned about both those possibilities. In addition, he said that when he performed abdominal surgery after a recurrence, he would usually find an abdomen full of cancer "like splattered mud." That was not

Micki's condition. On a short-term basis, we took his comments as positive signs. We knew that there would be further recurrences. There would no longer be any talk of a cure. For the time being, however, it seemed that the results of the surgery were the best we could have hoped for under the circumstances. Micki would proceed with further chemotherapy as soon as she was sufficiently strong.

In retrospect, I can see there was a great difference in patient care between Micki's initial hospitalization in 2003 and her later hospitalization in 2009. Yale–New Haven Hospital, from our viewpoint, had undergone a total transition. In 2003, the rooms were dirty, the staff was unhappy, and the care was barely adequate, even though the doctors and nurses were excellent. The head of the hospital at that time was not popular, and that unhappiness was reflected everywhere. In 2009, a new leader had assumed the helm, and her attitude and competency were reflected in the great improvement in patient care. The rooms were clean, the staff was polite, and services had expanded substantially. As with the proverbial fish, everything comes from the head.

After six days at Yale–New Haven, Micki was moved to Gaylord Hospital. She had substantial pain, a high sugar level, and a poorly functioning lymph system. Gaylord had a step-down unit for medically complex patients who were well enough to be moved from an acute care hospital, but not sufficiently well to go home or be moved to a skilled nursing facility.

. . .

On February 25, Micki felt a lump in her neck. A CT scan was taken of her abdomen and neck, but the results were inconclusive. We were told that we would need to wait for a consultation with Tom Rutherford, which was scheduled for March 4. While we waited, and while our anxiety level grew, the mass in Micki's neck began to recede. By the time we saw Dr. Rutherford, it had disappeared. The medical consensus was that the lump had been a backup of the lymph system. Still, our lives were controlled by reactions to every lump or pain, transient or permanent. It was a terrible way to live.

Chapter 9

The Last Best Treatment

Chemotherapy was scheduled to start at the end of February. Tom Rutherford's office was involved in a trial utilizing Avastin, a drug that had shown some promise for delaying the spread of breast cancer but had not been approved for the treatment of ovarian cancer. The premise was that the drug would cut off the supply of oxygen to any malignant tumors, causing the tumors to die. If we elected to have an infusion of Avastin outside of the trial, the cost of more than $20,000 per infusion would not be covered by insurance. Fortunately, Micki was included in the trial, and Medicare assumed responsibility for the payment of the drug. In the seesaw world that is cancer treatment, we were excited about the possibilities.

Chemotherapy began at the end of February 2009, using Avastin and another drug. The schedule called for two weekly infusions of chemotherapy followed by one week to recuperate. Micki was scheduled to have six cycles. The treatment would continue well into June. We were warned of three potential side effects: nausea, increased blood pressure, and increased fatigue. The side effects could be cumulative.

Within a few days of each infusion, Micki experienced nausea, but it was generally controlled by medication. After each dose of chemotherapy, she would spend two days in bed. With each cycle, the fatigue increased. Limited by her stamina, we tried to reach some normality in our lives. We looked forward to the weekends of the first two weeks of each cycle and the third full week, when she received no chemotherapy.

Intermittently, when she had sufficient strength, Micki completed her thesis and submitted it for approval. She was aided greatly by her colleague, Yukiko Tonoike, and by her mentor, Frank Hole. If there was one person who was responsible for Micki's enrolling in the graduate program at Yale, it was Frank Hole. His knowledge of archaeology stimulated Micki. Later, when her spirits and stamina were at a low ebb, he urged her to continue toward her degree.

Likewise, Micki and Yukiko had formed a symbiotic relationship during their years together at Yale. Yukiko was a bright and enthusiastic archaeologist who was completing her PhD. A generation younger than Micki, she had a young baby and was married to a Turkish citizen who spent a great deal of time in Turkey. Yukiko had no family in the United States, and Micki treated her like a daughter, offering advice, admiration, and many meals at our house.

I had no illusions about the nature of the new treatment; at best, we were attempting to hold off a further decline as long as possible. Micki did not complain, although her outlook had changed considerably. While in 2003 she had seemed almost ambivalent about her chemotherapy, unsure that it would help, now she was willing to try any medication so long as there was a chance to buy time and so long as she retained some quality of life. After all, she wanted to reach two important goals in the next three months of 2009: going to Zoe's Bat Mitzvah on May 16 and getting her degree from Yale on May 26. With the aid of the oncology nurses, we timed Micki's chemotherapy so that she would have several days to recuperate before each event.

• • •

May 16, 2009, was a beautiful day. Zoe celebrated her Bat Mitzvah after more than a year of study and preparation. A Bat Mitzvah is an important life cycle event in any Jewish family, but it held additional meaning for our family. Ever since Micki had been first diagnosed with cancer, some six years earlier, she had wanted to live long enough to forge a lasting bond with our two grandchildren. When she suffered a recurrence, she set her own goal of living the four months until Zoe's Bat Mitzvah.

Micki had had a chemotherapy infusion on May 4. She had spent the next few days in bed, but was ready to witness Zoe and her rite of passage by the end of the following week. Micki looked sparkling. All of our friends who attended knew that she was in the middle of chemotherapy, but everyone marveled at the way she looked. As long as I had known Micki, she had refused to be seen in public without at least some makeup, her hair cut and brushed, and her clothing stylish. As sick as she was, she was determined not to look weak or ill at Zoe's Bat Mitzvah. She was not going to be Micki "the patient." Following the Saturday service and luncheon, Micki went home and was exhausted. She was too tired to attend a family gathering that night at David's house, but she had attained one of her goals. At the age of 13, Zoe was a mature young lady. She had spent a great deal of time with Micki throughout her illness, and Micki knew that she would always hold a place in Zoe's heart.

• • •

Traditionally, Yale awards its degrees on a Monday. Graduation was scheduled for May 26. Micki's thesis had been read and approved by two professors in the Department of Archaeology, the last step leading to her master's degree. She had distinguished herself with her scholarship and had earned the distinction of being the oldest graduate student at Yale to earn a degree in 2009! To add to her achievement, she had finished her thesis and was awarded her degree while in the midst of chemotherapy.

On May 25, I had arranged to surprise Micki by having a private dinner in her honor at our favorite restaurant. Fortunately, we had scheduled her infusions so that the graduation occurred at the end of a week's break from chemotherapy. We thought that would give her the best chance of making it through the weekend. In order to get her to go to the restaurant, I told her that we were celebrating her degree with David and our grandchildren. About 30 of our best friends and our immediate family greeted Micki as she entered the restaurant. Everyone was aware of her declining health. It would have been an achievement for any person over the age of 60 to return to school and obtain an advanced degree at Yale. Considering the circumstances, the milestone was even more remarkable. Frank Hole, Micki's mentor, described the years of work that had been involved in obtaining the degree. He spoke of the persistence that had characterized Micki's effort. I was the last one to speak, and I described her achievement as a triumph of courage. It was an incredibly emotional afternoon.

The next day, Micki was determined to march with the procession of graduates into the campus. It was a walk of a few blocks, and I was not sure that she would be able to make it. A few days earlier, I had contacted the secretary of the university. She had provided us with special police clearance to park as close as possible, so we passed through barricades to get to our reserved space. The secretary had also given us graduation tickets so that our family could sit close to Micki. We all cheered as she entered the campus and received her diploma. It was a perfect event for Micki. She smiled all weekend and was very proud that she had attained a long-sought goal. Yet it was a bittersweet weekend for those of us who were close to her.

• • •

Micki resumed chemotherapy. At one of her sessions, in the middle of June, the oncology nurses noticed that Micki's blood pressure had risen to an unusually high level during the course of the infusion. We had been warned that one of the side effects from Avastin, her chemotherapy drug, was elevated blood pressure. We were told that it "only occurred in a small percentage of patients"—a familiar refrain. Blood pressure medication was administered. Her blood pressure decreased, and we were advised to check it at home over the next several hours. Micki's medical history had never involved high blood pressure.

That night, I took Micki's blood pressure at about 10:00 p.m. It read 204/190 (much higher than the normal reading of about 120/80). Increased blood pressure generally does not cause a change in appearance, but she was beginning to become unresponsive. I took it again. It read 204/194. I called her internist's answering machine and left a message, and then I called an ambulance. Micki was taken to the Emergency Room at Yale–New Haven Hospital, and I followed in my car.

When I saw Micki in the emergency room, she was incoherent. It was difficult for her to respond to commands. The ER staff administered more blood pressure medication. I stayed with her through the night, and David joined me early in the morning when Micki was still in the emergency room. I decided to take advantage of David's presence and go outside to get some fresh air. As I walked away from the hospital, David called me on my cell phone and asked me to return immediately because Micki had suffered a seizure. At that point, she was not responding at all; shortly thereafter she went into a coma. David and I did not know if she would survive. The medical staff was focused on lowering her blood pressure and told us nothing about her prognosis. They were concerned about bleeding in the brain.

After a few hours, Micki's internist, Dr. Robert Henry, arrived. The hospital was having difficulty finding an empty bed, but Dr. Henry was not satisfied with the hospital's response. Eventually, he was able to pressure the staff to locate a bed in intensive care. Micki was still unconscious as she was moved out of the ER.

For a few days, Micki remained in a coma. Gradually, her blood pressure was lowered by medication, but it was far from normal. There seemed to be an emerging medical consensus that the sudden elevation was a side effect of the Avastin. At that time, no one was concerned about her cancer, however. There was a more immediate problem: saving her life.

I was at the hospital continually. Micki's problem was neurological, so I had immediately contacted the best neurologist I knew—my brother, Fred. There was never a question in his mind that the episode was related to the Avastin. He was in Maryland, but he talked to a few of Micki's doctors and assured me that she would emerge from the coma, but that it would take time.

During the second day, one of the doctors told me that if Micki emerged from the coma, she might be permanently blind. My father had ended up with a loss of sight during his final hospital stay, many years ago. Although there was no similarity between his condition and Micki's, the mere thought of blindness panicked me. If I had to add the loss of sight to Micki's poor cancer prognosis, I began to wonder if she would be better off not surviving. This was not the last time that I would weigh quality-of-life issues against her survival.

I called my brother. He assured me that she was not going to be blind, but he thought that she might have some speech difficulties, which could be frustrating and require speech therapy. Learning this, I immediately asked for and received a change in the doctor who was caring for Micki.

• • •

About two days later, at 6:00 a.m., Micki was again visited by her internist, Dr. Henry. He tried to elicit a response from Micki by asking her a question. Surprisingly, she opened her eyes and answered him! She had emerged from her coma. My brother came to visit her the next day, by which time she was speaking a few words at a time. Her speech was halting, but clear. Over the next few days, her speech returned to normal. She would not need speech therapy, although she did need physical therapy to help her get back some of the strength that she had lost. Her blood pressure came back to near normal, although she would take blood pressure medication for the rest of her life. She would also be followed regularly by a cardiologist. After several more days, Micki returned home.

Micki did not remember most of the details of the hospitalization, including her ambulance ride, time in the emergency room, and early recovery. She recalled only the last two days.

I was glad that she was no longer in the hospital. However, from that time forward, I was concerned about rapid rises in her blood pressure. She and I constantly monitored her readings. On a few occasions, I called the doctor when I became alarmed about higher numbers. It was clear that I was overreacting. It was another instance in which I, in effect, was drawn into the middle of a storm and could not escape. What affected Micki also affected me. We were inextricably bound together.

As a result of this episode, Micki's chemotherapy schedule had been disrupted and delayed. It was resumed, without Avastin, within a few weeks.

Chapter 10

The Long Downward Spiral

Our life together was driven by the chemotherapy treatment schedule. During the "off week" in the three-week cycle, we had more of an opportunity to try to reconnect with our friends. I had forgotten what my daily life was like before Micki's recurrence: swimming or playing tennis a few times a week; attending lectures or taking a course at Yale during the week; a social life that was marked by our going to dinner with our friends frequently and to lunch with my friends regularly; a movie a few times a month; vacations each year. Those carefree days seemed long ago. I was now in a tunnel, and my vision of life around me was restricted by very narrow walls.

The presence of cancer in ovarian cancer patients can be detected in three ways: a physical examination, a CT scan or other diagnostic radiology, or a blood test to determine a CA-125 reading. When Micki was diagnosed in 2003, she did not register on the CA-125 scale. Apparently, that failure to register occurs in about 15 percent of ovarian cancer patients.

In almost all cases, however, even those patients demonstrate a reading when a recurrence happens. That was Micki's experience.

A normal CA-125 is below 35. While she was receiving chemotherapy, Micki's CA-125 was in the 50 to 70 range. Although some oncologists may not consider that reading to be unusually high, it is not low enough for the patient to be considered in remission. Micki's physical examinations continued to be normal, and, at the end of the scheduled course of chemotherapy, her CA-125 was in the 10 to 12 range. This indicated to me that she was in remission. We were pleased about her perceived progress.

Tom Rutherford scheduled another CT scan, to be followed by an appointment with him to discuss the results. We arrived at his office for a 2:45 p.m. appointment on December 30, 2009. While we waited, we noticed that many people who had arrived after us had been seen and left. I took this as a bad sign. Finally, when we were ushered into his office, he told us that the CT scan had shown a spread of the ovarian cancer to Micki's liver and lungs. Rather than remission, minute cells, too many and too small for surgery, were proliferating. Tom was very upset with the results and said that Micki would need another course of chemotherapy. This course would last for 18 weeks, and, hopefully, put her back in remission. If not, there were many more poisons to try, all with the increased possibility of greater side effects and with the diminishing possibility of attaining even a temporary remission.

The news was devastating. I held no illusions about the possible success of the next round of drugs. I had had a discussion with one of Tom's colleagues several months earlier, and he had told me that after a recurrence, the chance of getting back into remission becomes less and less, as each course of chemotherapy fails. I did not repeat that conversation to Micki. She had completed three different protocols since her recurrence and surgery, all without success. We were starting with the fourth.

There was no disguising Tom's disappointment. To us, he was not the distant and efficient surgeon, void of personality. He was our friend and confidant. We had placed our faith in his hands. We had a mutual stake in the never-ending struggle.

• • •

It had been 39 years since Richard Nixon had announced a war on cancer. Now, after all that time has passed, nearly 600,000 Americans still die each year from cancer. One in three women and one in two men still experience cancer during their lifetimes. The fruits of research allow some cancer victims to live longer. On the other hand, the longevity of the general population means that more cancers are diagnosed. While some types of cancer now have improved cure rates, the overall incidence of cancer has not declined.

Cancer is caused by the uncontrolled proliferation of cells. Tom Rutherford told us that the Yale Cancer Center had been able to identify Micki's aberrant cell—unfortunately, it was a stem cell and could not be killed. Science, in 39 years, appeared to have arrived at the cause of most cancers and could even isolate the killer cell, but it could not destroy it. So near and yet so far. The next leap, the ability to kill the aberrant cell, would occur long after that giant step could save Micki's life.

• • •

In retrospect, I realize that I was starting my own grieving process at about this time. Clearly, with the discovery that cancer had recurred and spread at the beginning of 2009, our hopes for a cure were all but gone. For the rest of the year, Micki took all the medical treatment that was offered to her with the goal of remission and the hopes of treating the disease as a chronic illness and adding to her borrowed time.

By the end of 2009, in my heart, I felt that even a compromised life of several years was not likely. I did not share my feelings with Micki. I did not know if she was ready to accept an imminent death. Tom, the true warrior, certainly did not accept the immediacy of her death. Even though the odds favoring remission grew slimmer with each new protocol, he was willing to roll the dice. Tom Rutherford was a perfectionist, an ardent advocate for his patients, and a trusted friend. It was not for me to intercede. I owed it to Micki to make the best of a bad situation. I had been her cheerleader until now, and I was determined not to relinquish that role.

Now, rather than feeling the distant cloud hanging over our heads, I felt the cloud was finally descending on us. We vowed to each other that we would do our best to make every day count. David, in particular, talked to Micki about putting meaning into every day. David and I suggested to Micki that she have some discussions with a therapist, and David suggested that I do the same. I talked with a psychologist about my feelings in January 2010. I chose not to continue therapy at that time, but we agreed to meet as I felt the need. Micki preferred to face her problems alone. She enlarged her tight circle of friends slightly, but did not discuss any of her concerns about her illness with them.

Micki and I each had our own circle of friends and also couples that we saw together. We started going out for dinner or a movie with friends when Micki felt strong enough. Sometimes we simply took a long ride together. Those plans were always subject to a last-minute cancellation if Micki was not feeling well, because her strength was difficult to predict on any given day.

Separately, I saw my own friends for lunch or to play tennis but much less frequently than I had before Micki suffered her recurrence. As I was getting very depressed at home, I looked forward to getting out. However, each time I left the house, I felt guilty. I thought that I should be spending that time with Micki. Who knew how many days we had left together? I lived with the guilt and frustration of helplessness.

Micki was heroic. She never asked, "Why me?" She didn't complain. She accepted the facts as they were. She knew that we were constantly inquiring about possible new treatments. She had complete faith in Tom Rutherford. He assured me that the Yale Cancer Center was in a network of the best cancer centers in the country and that he was always looking for potential new treatments. Micki was intent on controlling the environment around her. She took pride in making cosmetic changes to our house, saying, "It will be ready for Ed when I am no longer here." What she could not control, she left to her doctors.

Micki was determined to leave me, David, and our grandchildren with the feeling that she had done everything possible to provide for our future. She and I spent a lot of time discussing the gift that we had received by her surviving for the last six years. We had accomplished a lot together.

David was a wonderful father, successful in his profession, and had established a long-term relationship with Katie. Our grandchildren had grown from young children of nine and six years to young teens. We enjoyed a close and loving relationship with them. In the interim, Micki had undergone four surgeries and innumerable courses of chemotherapy. She had been able to continue her studies and receive her degree. Had Micki died shortly after her initial diagnosis, she would have missed these blessings.

• • •

As Micki's health worsened and she became weaker, our conversations were filled with reminiscences of our life together. We recounted the early days of our relationship and the questions that casual onlookers had raised about our marriage. We had heard about their comments after the fact. After 39 years, Micki and I had the last laugh. At the onset, we heard that people wondered if I had married Micki because of her physical beauty, or if she had married me because I was a lawyer and "had some money." Superficially, we appeared to be so different. We spent some time exploring the real reasons for our marriage.

In fact, I had married Micki because of her courage, her determination, and her intelligence. Those characteristics were much more important to me than the superficial quality of beauty. I was aware of the problems that Micki had lived through with her family and the difficulties she faced as a single parent bringing up David. She had persevered. Courage, determination, and intelligence were enduring qualities. The way she faced her final illness put those qualities to the test. In a very intimate moment, I told her that she was my hero—she was the most courageous person I had ever known.

She told me that she was drawn to me by my inner strength. Many times she had said that I was the most secure person she had met. In her world of turmoil that preceded our dating, she craved security for herself and for David, and she felt that she had found it in our marriage.

Certainly, she knew that she was not marrying me for my wealth. Although I was a partner in a small law firm, I spent many hours each week in community service, not practicing law. Working in the community gave me personal satisfaction, but not much money in my pocket. In the long run, I hoped that community involvement would help me develop my law practice. At the time of our marriage in 1971, however, and faced with the challenge of supporting a new family, my earnings had not exceeded $18,000 in any given year. I had no inherited assets and very little in the bank.

We had married because we truly loved each other, and that love had continued throughout our marriage. Those who speculated about other reasons for our marriage were no longer our friends.

We were intellectually compatible. For many years of our years together, we had developed the habit of watching the evening news as we were eating dinner together. In the beginning, when David was eating with us, the news served as a vehicle to encourage discussions among us and as a teaching tool for our son. After David left home for college, Micki and I continued our routine. I was addicted to current events and politics. Where I looked at a news event of the day with excitement and for its history-making significance, Micki's archaeological training led her to look at the same event as a mere blip on a long arc of history, perhaps to be repeated at another time or in another civilization. She read constantly, and we had endless discussions about the effect of the past upon the present.

Gradually, as she became weaker, her interest in the world around her lessened. I knew that her mind was elsewhere when Osama Bin Laden was killed. I received almost no reaction when I told her the news.

Even as her interests narrowed, Micki never tired of hearing about our grandchildren. We spent time talking about their futures. We both wanted to leave them with a legacy. I don't know if she realized that her strength in facing death was part of that legacy. Many times, I told Micki that we should be thankful for her years of remission, as that period had established her relationship with them.

In the last several weeks of her life, it was difficult for Micki to sustain a conversation. In the last two weeks, she did not talk at all. Throughout her illness, Micki wanted to talk about life, not death. It was up to her to set the boundaries.

By the end of 2009, Micki had accepted the fact that she was dying, but she was not ready to accept when she would die. Neither was I. Even if she did not attain a remission, we could not, at that stage, predict the remaining length of her life. In the meantime, the repetitive chemical infusions were taking a physical toll. Despite good intentions and promises to each other that we would make the most of each remaining day, the thought of her death dominated our lives. It was difficult to smile. It was painful to laugh.

On one occasion, Micki sensed my depression, even though I did my best to hide it from her. She told me that she wanted me to emerge from our life together as a husband who was still intact. We had a pistol in the house. She said that, if her condition was overwhelming me, she was prepared to use the pistol to end her life. I assured her that, as far as I was concerned, taking her own life was not an option. That conversation was never repeated.

• • •

In August 2010, we paid a monthly visit to Tom Ruther-ford. For a few days, Micki had been feeling better and had more energy. We grasped at any straw as a hopeful sign. He deflated our feelings by telling us that her CA-125 numbers had increased and suggested that she felt better because of a change in the chemotherapy. The rise in the CA-125 was a sign that the cancer was spreading. I asked him about our options. He said that Micki might be able to participate in a new trial that his group was trying to put together. It would take several months before the trial could begin. From the look on Tom's face, I was not sure that Micki would be alive long enough to participate.

• • •

Micki continued to have chemotherapy throughout 2010. In the fall of that year, I woke up one morning and looked across the bed at her. She was lying on her back, look-ing at the ceiling. I realized that I was really suffering. Not because she was dying and I would miss her—I had come to accept that inevitability—and not because I had fears about what would happen to me after she was gone—to the extent that my health was reasonably good, I thought I would be able to carve a new life. Instead, I was hurting because I was watching Micki suffer and it was so painful for me to observe. My love for her had not diminished. She had, long ago, lost many vestiges of her former self. She had expressed this to me when she lost her ovaries, then when sex lost its meaning and when she lost her hair. She was, above all, determined not to complain as she was dying. This determination was harder to achieve as her body failed her. She hoped that she had been a role model for her son and grandchildren. Now, at the end of her life, she was determined to be a role model in facing death with dignity.

At the end of 2010, Micki had come face-to-face with trying to survive for one day longer each day . . . and each day was getting shorter. Her weakness was apparent each time she tried to climb the stairs to our bedroom. She stayed in bed almost all day—partly because she was tired all the time and partly because she no longer had the energy or lung capacity to climb the stairs. She rarely smiled, usually maintaining a frown and a look of deep concentration. Still, she did not let me into her world. It was as if she wanted to protect me from a world of despair.

Micki was locked in a struggle of life and death, and she knew she wasn't winning. It had to be terrifying. The most I could do was to make her comfortable and put my arms around her. Sometimes, I would cross the hallway to our den, my eyes overflowing. That was my suffering. I didn't verbalize it to Micki. To describe it would have been too devastating for her. The torturous path Micki was taking to death was sacred ground. It was simply too painful or too cruel a subject to broach.

Each time we visited Tom Rutherford, we asked about the trial that he had mentioned. We looked on it as a long shot but as our last hope to reduce the growth of the cancer. A potential approval date for the trial had been postponed because further work was required.

• • •

The last half of 2010 was marked by several hospitalizations. Usually, they were caused by a fever. Thanks to chemotherapy, Micki's body was incapable of fighting any infection. Toward the end of the year, we were caught in a revolving door of chemotherapy that did not work and trips to the hospital whenever Micki's temperature exceeded 101 degrees. There was no hope that her condition would improve. It was exhausting, physically and mentally, for both of us.

We spent our anniversary, December 12, 2010, in the hospital. By the time the new year began, Micki was back in the hospital again. By that time, a large tumor was pressing against her lung, causing the lung to partially collapse. Her breathing was severely restricted, and her condition had deteriorated so substantially that she would not qualify for the trial, if it was ever approved.

At the end of the January hospitalization, Tom Rutherford was intent on starting a new course of chemotherapy.

He was a fighter who simply did not want to concede. However, during Micki's hospitalization I had started conversations with two other doctors. The first was Micki's original oncologist, Arthur Levy, who had left private practice and was working as a clinical oncologist at Yale–New Haven Hospital. We met by accident at a coffee counter in the hospital. We shared coffee and talked about Micki's diminished quality of life and our future direction. He was helping me face the next step. Arthur told me that he thought Tom would talk to Micki soon about the viability of further chemotherapy. I felt that the scale was tipping and that Micki's suffering was beginning to outweigh any pleasure that could be gained by extending her life. Once again, though, I was reduced to the role of helpless onlooker. Any decision about discontinuing treatment would be made by Micki.

The tumor that had compromised Micki's breathing was full of fluid. In order to alleviate some pressure on her lung, it was necessary to insert a tube into the tumor and begin to drain the fluid. That procedure, if successful, would allow the lung to expand. As I returned to Micki's room, she was undergoing the drainage procedure.

When I reached her floor, I was greeted by Dr. Larry Solomon, who had been Micki's internist when she was starting graduate school. He was currently serving as the head of palliative care at the Yale Cancer Center. Larry was thoroughly familiar with Micki's medical record and knew that there was no hope for any kind of recovery. He told me that we needed to think about hospice. His recommendation came as no surprise. I had been living with Micki's deterioration for so long that nothing would have surprised me. I asked him to discuss her treatment with Tom Rutherford.

That night, when Tom visited Micki, she asked him if further chemotherapy was going to help her condition. He admitted that it was not likely. I wish I had been with Micki at the time. Unfortunately, I did not know that Tom was going to see her, and I had gone home for the evening. She was left to ask the difficult question alone.

I know it was very difficult for Tom to admit to Micki that he could no longer help her. He was a supreme advocate for his patients. He was the doctor who you wanted in your corner *when you had a chance to survive.* Unfortunately, we were beyond that point. Micki told me that, when he admitted that further treatment would not benefit her, they cried together. Tom sent me a message expressing his regret that he could not do more for Micki, saying that he had great respect for her and referring to her as a "wonderful lady."

We had to face the essential question: where does the dedication to prolonging life end and a concern for the quality and dignity of remaining life prevail?

Micki and I had a brief but very painful conversation. We agreed that there was nothing further to be gained by more chemotherapy. I spent all that morning holding Micki's hand. With the help of compassionate doctors, we made a choice in favor of her quality of life. The time for injecting poison into Micki's system every few weeks and living a life ruled by the side effects of chemotherapy was over. Realistically, I knew that Micki's time was very limited. I wanted her to live out her remaining days with as much comfort and dignity as possible. I told her that I only wanted her not to suffer.

In her final days, palliative care and hospice played a major role in reducing Micki's suffering. While she was receiving chemotherapy and getting progressively weaker, Micki had received care through Hospice's CanSupport program, which is designed for people who cannot take complete care of themselves, yet may live for an indeterminate time. Through the CanSupport program, we were given a home health aide for several hours a week. We were also monitored closely by Michelle Avenia, a wonderful, caring nurse, who visited Micki at least every week. Hospice also offered emotional support as part of the program. Initially, Micki was willing to see a social worker; however, after a few weeks, Micki again rejected professional emotional support. She told me that she had nothing to discuss with the social worker. On the other hand, Micki welcomed the home health aide and nurse as she grew weaker and less able to care for herself.

. . .

Micki had been placed on oxygen as soon as she entered the hospital at the end of 2010. In January 2011, when the drain was inserted into her lung, we had hoped that her oxygen dependency would decrease, but she still required the full-time use of oxygen when she was discharged. Hoping that she would gain some strength and be able to breathe without the oxygen, Micki went to Gaylord Hospital for a few weeks of physical therapy. It helped: she regained her balance and was walking with some regularity.

Still, Micki's difficulty with breathing continued. A diagnostic X-ray determined that the drainage tube was no longer working. Although most of the fluid had been cleared from the tumor, it continued to grow and was still constricting her lung. Because of Micki's weakened condition and the advanced state of her disease, it was decided that no further interventions would be undertaken. Instead, she would remain on oxygen for her remaining life.

Chapter 11

Final Months

Micki came home on February 1, 2011. She was comfortable in her own bed, looking out the window at a peaceful scene of lawn, trees, and a river at the edge of our property. Once we made the decision to terminate chemotherapy, the frequency of Micki's care increased as she transitioned to the outpatient hospice program.

When Micki left the hospital, I asked Tom Rutherford about her projected life expectancy. He told me that he thought she would live for another three to five months. Micki was unaware of our conversation.

At some point, death passed from becoming an abstract concept to a reality. Death had truly taken on a life of its own. When you are told that your spouse probably has three to five months to live, if you are the primary caregiver, there are certain choices to be made.

Hospice had suggested that we set up a hospital bed in

our room, next to the bed that Micki and I shared. Michelle, our hospice nurse, thought that it would be easier for Micki to get in and out of the hospital bed. Although Michelle did not say this to Micki, the hospital bed also would have made it easier for the health aides to lift and turn Micki when she was unable to do it for herself. It became a moot point when Micki rejected the bed. She was against any outward sign of illness and dependency. For Micki, to move to a hospital bed would have been an admission that she was one step closer to death. For nearly 40 years, I had slept in the same bed with her, and she did not want to change that pattern or disrupt the routine of normality that was so important to her. She knew that death was unavoidable, but she wanted to do everything in her power to push back the timetable.

• • •

While Micki already had succeeded in establishing a bond with Joshua and Zoe, she felt a need to leave them a material legacy. Although Zoe was then only 14, she had reached a height that enabled her to wear some of Micki's clothes. Micki encouraged Zoe to try them on. Of course, this was difficult for Zoe emotionally, because it was a sign that she was going to lose her grandmother. Micki and I also agreed that Zoe would inherit all of Micki's jewelry. They spent hours together, as Micki described each piece in detail to Zoe.

After discussing it with David, Micki and I let Joshua know that he would receive our collection of ancient pottery from Israel after we both had died. Joshua, at the age of 17, was also an excellent photographer, and for a few months in 2010, he and Micki had met each week to write an historical description of each piece of pottery, photograph it, and compile a catalogue.

Micki was building her legacy and preserving a sense of continuity. That was very important to her.

Carefully, I picked a moment to discuss Micki's future care with her. We both rejected the thought of a skilled nursing facility. I would coordinate her home care, regardless of the cost, until the last few days, when she suggested that she would move to the inpatient hospice facility. I didn't realize that the health aides provided by hospice, at our home, would be adequate until the last few weeks of her life and were also fully covered by Medicare. Although I interviewed a home health agency to supplement the hospice personnel, we did not need additional help until the very end.

• • •

On February 25, 2011, as Micki was being cared for by a home health aide, she collapsed. She was breathing normally, but was not responsive. I was at home and was immediately able to reach Michelle, our hospice nurse, who was in the area. When Michelle arrived, Micki was still unresponsive, but her vital signs were normal. Micki began to stir as Michelle talked to her, but she could not talk. Her ability to follow commands was limited.

Michelle told me that we had three choices: (1) we could leave Micki at home and see if she responded, (2) we could take her by ambulance to Yale–New Haven Hospital, or (3) we could take her by ambulance to the hospice inpatient facility. Michelle thought that Micki had either suffered a small stroke or that the cancer had spread to her brain. In either case, it made no sense to do further diagnostic testing because her death was unavoidable and imminent. If Micki went to Yale–New Haven Hospital, because she was no longer on chemotherapy, she would have to be admitted through the emergency room. At most acute care facilities, patients are treated as if they are part of a herd when they come to the ER. Yale was no different, and I felt that Micki had been through too much to subject her to that charged environment. On the other hand, if Micki went to hospice and recovered, she would be observed for a few days and then brought back home. Since I had heard only good things about hospice treatment, and we had planned to move Micki there to die, I thought it made more sense for her to be transported to the hospice facility for observation and for any treatment that was required.

Micki began to respond as soon as she arrived at hospice.

The building was the former headquarters of a major corpo-
ration and sat on the edge of Long Island Sound. Each patient
room had a view of the water. However, for financial effi-
ciency and ease of care, each room contained three or four
patient beds; there was virtually no privacy. Micki was 71.
Although she was deteriorating physically, her deterioration
was slow, and she was very alert mentally. When she woke up
in her room and looked around her, she saw three other
women, each 20 years older than she was, and all within two
or three days of death. The setting was depressing, which was
not the fault of hospice. It was a function of the terminal status of the patients. Fortunately, Micki recovered quickly and
wanted to return home immediately. She was well enough to
be transported back there within a few days.

As a result of her hospice inpatient experience, Micki
and I promised each other that she would die at home.
Although that decision might place more of a burden on me,
it was the least that I could do for my wife. We would be
together until the end.

• • •

The months of March, April, and May were relatively
uneventful—which is not to say that they were marked by a
normal way of life. It was virtually impossible for Micki to
come downstairs. She was tethered to a long oxygen line. The

health aide came every day and helped her into the shower and made breakfast. I made all her lunches and dinners.

I felt that I should be with Micki as much as possible. The strain that we were both under was affecting me, though, and I was in desperate need of a daily break. When Micki slept or had company, I would go into the den to read or watch a basketball game. When a home health aide was with her, I would find it a luxury to drive to the grocery store. There were times when I would prolong the trip. I would take a detour on my way home, so long as I knew an aide was with Micki. Anything to take advantage of a temporary lifting of the cloud that hovered over us every day.

Micki was still able to get out of bed and walk to the bathroom—a distance of about 25 feet—but her shortness of breath was so acute that she was required to stop for at least 30 seconds to gather her strength. One day she lost her balance in the bathroom and narrowly missed striking her head on the shower door. I was in the next room and came in when I heard her fall. She was undressed, lying helplessly on the floor, in a pool of urine. I could not lift her. She no longer had strength in her own legs. Together, we could not get her to more than a kneeling or sitting position. I was left with no alternative but to call for an EMT. Two paramedics arrived after several minutes. They helped her get on her feet and return to bed.

For a woman who had great pride and self-respect, this

was an embarrassing episode. By the time the EMTs had arrived, I had partially covered Micki with a bathrobe, but she was humiliated. From that time forward, we kept a portable commode next to the bed.

Micki had visits from her closest friends. On those occasions, she made sure that she was dressed, applied makeup, and walked (with her oxygen) out of the bedroom to visit with them in our den, which was located on the same floor. Her friend Sarah called from Florida at least once each week, sent cards regularly, and flew to Connecticut monthly to be with Micki. Micki's emotions were positive when she had company, but she would never ask anyone to visit, so I made arrangements for friends to come over. The highlight of each week was the weekend, when David and Katie spent time with us and were often joined by one or both of our grandchildren. Each week, Abby, David's former wife, would arrive with a container of soup and would visit with Micki.

During that period, I had an encounter with a relative who had been particularly close to us. When Micki began her final decline, our relative would email me asking about Micki. At the time, there were very few people Micki wanted to see, but this relative was one of them. After her many promises that she would "be in touch in a few days to arrange for a visit," I decided to confront her. At the risk of our friendship, I asked if she was simply afraid to visit a woman who was dying. She hesitated before responding and tried to change the subject. She was clearly embarrassed. I told her that, except for her oxygen, Micki appeared normal. She was alert, looked good, and wanted to see her. The relative came to our house in a few days, had a good visit with Micki, and thanked me for intervening.

One day, my friend Tom Corradino came to my home so that we could have a sandwich on our patio. Tom asked me if all of Micki's medical expenses were covered by insurance. Before I could answer him, he added, "Because if they are not covered, I will write you a check." And he meant it. Tom had a heart full of kindness. It was as big as the world.

For many families who must deal with a cancer situation, money does not become an issue. For patients who are covered by Medicare, a Medigap policy, and, eventually, inpatient or outpatient hospice care, almost all medical costs are covered, including chemotherapy and medications. Once a patient is under the hospice umbrella, nursing care, home health aides, and drugs are also covered. The only major expense is for additional home care, over and above that provided by hospice or a private insurance policy. In our particular situation, through all of Micki's illness, our out-of-pocket expenses did not exceed $3,000. Fortunately, I was not working and was available as a major caregiver, so even when Micki was able to care for herself, she was not alone.

My friends remained true. Several of them called

regularly and asked if they could do anything. A few became regular companions at lunch, and I depended on them to give me an hour of respite. Micki could not be left alone, so my hour away usually coincided with a visit by a friend of Micki's or a daily visit by the home health aide. There were also times when I was scheduled to see friends and cancelled at the last minute because of Micki's needs.

David Lesser was a friend whom I relied upon increasingly. He and I were both lawyers who had become disenchanted with the practice of law. I retired and went back to school. David retired and became a rare book dealer. I could speak candidly with David about feelings of depression and guilt. He listened and never lectured. On the other hand, we could also become involved in a lively debate about politics. He was patient and more than willing to adjust his agenda to my concerns. He lent me a sympathetic ear when I needed it the most.

One night, I arranged to have our friend Lynn Cadan visit with Micki while I went out to our favorite restaurant with her husband, Alan, for a leisurely dinner. It was the first time that I had been out in many months. I found that I was nearly euphoric with my taste of freedom.

I had also begun to look forward to trips to the grocery store several times each week as a break in my routine and a chance to breathe some fresh air. Each of those excursions, however, brought an overwhelming feeling of guilt. How could I enjoy myself, for even a few minutes, while my wife was dying?

When I was at home, it was obvious to me that Micki wanted me near her. It was not that we engaged in deep conversations. In fact, she avoided many of those conversations because she felt they would revolve around her declining health. She just wanted me to be physically close. After a 39-year marriage, before she had suffered her recurrence of cancer, we frequently held hands. If I failed to sit next to her and hold her hand while she was sick, I was afraid that she would think that I was treating her like a pariah. We were still bound together.

Micki began to sleep more frequently—a sign that her body was weakening. When she fell asleep in the early evening, I would leave the bedroom and walk to the den to watch a baseball game on television. After some time, she would wake and call for me. When I realized that I was enjoying the solitude of watching television or reading, alone, I was overwhelmed with guilt.

The burden of care was wearing me down. On many days, I found that I could only look straight ahead and concentrate on putting one foot in front of the other. I felt as if I were carrying a 100-pound weight on my shoulders over a period of time. For the first several steps, I managed the burden. Over time, my shoulders drooped and ached. Then the pain spread through my core, as if the weight were pressing down on my spine, bone rubbing against bone. At some point numbness and tunnel vision took over. I moved ahead, slowly.

I hated the disease. Although I am somewhat ashamed to admit it, there were brief moments when I resented that Micki's death was taking so long. It was a cruel and selfish thought. Her death was inevitable. Why was she prolonging it? Fortunately, those moments were fleeting and were immediately followed by feelings of guilt.

More and more, I began to think of my life after Micki. One night, I remembered dreaming of lying on a beach with no one around me and nothing that I had to do. I had a big smile on my face. I woke up to reality.

I also had many bad dreams that someone I knew was sick or dying. The subject matter was not surprising. Sleep was not a respite.

So long as Micki was not in an acute situation and had care, David urged me to get out more frequently. I knew he was concerned for my well-being. I was pulled in two directions: I needed to regain some of my autonomy, but Micki had an emotional need to have me with her. I tried to put myself in her shoes. Although she never demonstrated her fear outwardly, I thought that she must have been scared to confront death alone. To the extent that I could lessen that fear by being with her, I needed to be there.

The guilt became a large part of my life, and I felt that

I needed to talk to someone about it. I arranged to talk with a psychologist and friend, who told me that my thoughts about freedom and my life after Micki were perfectly normal given the circumstances. Our conversation helped ease the burden—at least temporarily.

As before, I urged her to share her thoughts with a psychiatrist, a social worker, or our rabbi. She spoke to all of them once or twice after her recurrence, but ultimately rejected their offers of help. It may have been that she was in a state of denial. She did not want to say goodbye.

My friends formed a support group that pulled me up by the shoulders when I fell down. Our former and future daughters-in-law were with Micki constantly and helped me often. I had a caring son, who was grieving for his mother and was very concerned for me. They made an intolerable situation more livable, but they all went home at night. In the last few weeks of Micki's life, I knew that I would need to face her final journey by myself.

• • •

During the winter and spring of 2011, I had been preoccupied with my 50th college reunion. Talking to many of my classmates was a diversion for me, and, as a class officer, I worked to raise money for our class gift to Yale University. My friend Vince Teti was the Class Gift Chairman. Several months earlier, when Micki and I had met Vince and his wife for dinner, Vince had suggested creating a Class Initiative for the Yale Cancer Center as part of our reunion gift. We felt that the achievements and future of the Yale Cancer Center were very exciting and that many classmates would be attracted to that need. We knew that we could obtain contributions for the Cancer Center from some classmates who might not otherwise be inclined to give to the University at all. We were right. Although we started our specific campaign late in the reunion year and worked with a small committee, by June 1 we were able to raise $1.2 million for the Yale Cancer Center. I reported each gift to Micki, and this was a source of inspiration to her.

A few weeks before the reunion, I received a telephone call from my good friend and classmate Sherwin Goldman. Over the years, he and Micki had developed a particularly close friendship. Sherwin wanted to visit Micki; he knew that she was approaching the end, and, in essence, he wanted to say goodbye. I remember the two of them, sitting in our den, simply holding hands. I was overcome with emotion and needed to leave the room.

The reunion was scheduled to run from Thursday night through Saturday night in New Haven. I had not been separated from Micki for many months. I arranged for David and his fiancée, Katie, to stay with Micki while I was at the reunion, but I would be sleeping at home each night.

As the weekend approached, I kept thinking of Micki and decided not to attend some events so that I could spend more time with her. Micki had always attended class events with me over the years, and my classmates and their wives, many of whom knew of Micki's illness, were very thoughtful. I realized that I was having difficulty smiling. For me, it was a weekend of both pleasure and pain. While enjoying my reunion, I could not separate myself from my situation at home.

Sometime later, Katie told me about the conversations she had with Micki that weekend. Katie said that Micki knew the end was approaching. She had no regrets about her life. She was at peace with herself and with our long marriage. She said that she had picked the right father for David when she married me and was happy and proud of the relationship that David and I had forged. She felt that the last few years had given her the opportunity to help our grandchildren form their own identities, and she felt that they had absorbed some of our values and ideals. I, too, felt at peace when Katie described those conversations.

Chapter 12

Remember Me

As June progressed, Micki slept more and more. Her doctor had warned that, if she suffered a stomach blockage, which was not uncommon with abdominal cancers, she would need surgery to bypass the bowel. Micki was determined to avoid the surgery. She forced herself to eat, drink, and take medication, all in order to keep her digestive tract open. To require an external device to bypass the bowel would have been the ultimate humiliation for Micki. It would have represented her final loss of dignity. This was a battle she won.

On June 21, a palpable tumor could be felt in Micki's stomach. There was nothing that could be done about it. Her eating was slowing to a crawl. That day, she suffered another collapse and became unresponsive. Michelle, our nurse, felt that Micki's brain was affected. It was not a stroke. She slept more frequently. When she was awake, she smiled and could shake her head. She understood everything that was said to her, but she could not speak. She would never speak again.

There is one thing that can be said for most cancer deaths: the spouse and family have plenty of time to say goodbye. I spoke with Micki several times in the last few weeks. I reminded her of our long marriage and our love and devotion for each other. The last time I spoke with her was after she had lost the ability to respond verbally. I know that she heard me because she squeezed my hand.

Michelle felt that Micki should be taken to hospice to die. Based on our previous experience, I refused. Micki no longer had the strength to move from the bed to the commode, and she finally agreed to be moved to a hospital bed. We also arranged for her to have round-the-clock care. Michelle recommended Sharon Fraser, a home health aide. Sharon was a large and gentle woman who had no trouble moving Micki around. Sharon slept in my bed, next to the hospital bed, and I moved into the den. Sharon worked around the clock, relieved for a few hours each day when the regular hospice home health aide arrived. That aide and a nurse were now visiting daily.

I was in and out of the bedroom constantly. When Micki slept, I tried to get some solitude. When she was awake, I tried to be with her. By July 1, she was sleeping 90 percent of the time. She had stopped eating solid food and was consuming only ice and occasionally water.

I wasn't sure about the level of Micki's awareness. Watching her die was more painful for me than the thought of her not living. I remembered my conversation with Vince Teti several years earlier: I was not afraid of Micki's dying, I was afraid of getting there. Several days before, I had told the nurses that when she was approaching death, I wanted it to come quickly. I was only interested in avoiding suffering.

David was with us often, as were Katie and Abby. I thought about involving our grandchildren, but worried that seeing their grandmother close to death could be too traumatic. On the other hand, to have them with her would be an act of loving kindness. I left the choice to David and Abby. Within an hour, Joshua and Zoe were at Micki's bedside, holding her hand. The next morning, I asked Micki if she remembered that our grandchildren had visited her. She smiled and nodded. She was still aware.

• • •

On the morning of July 7, at about 5:00 a.m., I heard Sharon come down the hall to the den. She knocked on my door and told me that she thought Micki was dying. I went into the bedroom and saw that Micki was having trouble breathing and that her eyes were wide open. Her breathing was shallow and erratic. She was in distress. The hospice nurse lived close to our home and arrived quickly; she confirmed that Micki was dying and increased her medication to attempt to relieve any suffering. Once again, I was helpless.

I called David, and he came quickly. We spent the morning together. I had told myself that I was ready for Micki's death, but when it appeared to be near, I was concerned about having second thoughts. Still, I knew in my heart that it was time.

Hospice had called in another nurse, Sandra Johnson. She was a kind, elderly woman with a deep sense of the spiritual. She was used by hospice to deal with actual death situations. She and Sharon, who was standing by, said that they both felt that it was a calling to help an ill person pass out of this world with as much dignity and as little pain as possible. They were with Micki for the rest of the morning, keeping her clean and cool. They tried to calm her. To the extent that Micki looked agitated, Sandra assured us that Micki was not aware of any pain or discomfort. At about noon, there was a change in Micki's breathing pattern. Sandra turned to David and me and said, "She's passing over now. You can still talk to her."

Hospice had prepared us well. We knew that Micki had a level of consciousness until the end. It was our job to allow her to pass away peacefully. Separately, David and I each told Micki that we loved her. We said that she had been a wonderful wife and mother. We told her that her family was all right and she no longer had to worry about us.

Micki was still not ready to die. What had sustained her in life—her indomitable courage—made it more difficult for her to die. Her breathing was labored. Hospice had instructed us that in the end, we should tell the patient that she could let go. Neither David nor I could bring ourselves to do that. Neither of us wanted to be the one to say goodbye.

Katie arrived, and we told her about our reluctance. She went into the bedroom, put her arm around Micki, and told her that her family would be well. Then Katie told Micki that it was all right to let go. Micki took one long breath. A teardrop fell from one eye. And then it was over. Micki was gone. Her long journey had ended.

Robert Ruark, who wrote stirring novels about Africa, also wrote a semiautobiographical book at the end of his career, entitled *The Honey Badger*. He describes the honey badger as a ferocious and mean little animal that burrows its way into its victims and eats their innards. Ruark had his own honey badger. It was called prostate cancer. Micki, too, had a honey badger inside of her. For several years it had been eating away at her insides. Now, it had taken its toll. Only the blessing of modern medicine kept her from excruciating pain. She was barely clinging to life.

Micki succumbed to her honey badger. Its fangs reached out to those around her. I repelled the honey badger, but was forever scarred by its bite.

• • •

I had not opened the letter that Micki had written to me when she suffered her recurrence. Throughout her illness, she never asked me for anything. When I finally opened her letter, after she had died, it contained her final plea: REMEMBER ME.

Chapter 13

Climbing Out of the Abyss

Several weeks before Micki died, she designated the people that she wanted as her pallbearers. She wanted young people, not anyone in our generation. When I asked her why she had designated all young people, she said, "Because they are the future. They are the link between what has been and what will be. We can't live in the past." She picked our grandchildren, Abby, Katie, and our two nieces.

A few days before Micki died, when she had continual care and was sleeping almost all of the time, I went to New Haven and met with the funeral director to make arrangements for the funeral. I set up a group in my email address book so that a wide circle of friends would know that Micki had died and would be aware of the pending funeral. I also set up a phone network of our closest friends and relatives.

I wrote Micki's obituary and prepared her eulogy. I knew that I would be unable to read it at the funeral and asked the rabbi to do so. Micki and I had discussed other speakers for her funeral. In addition to David, Micki requested that Sarah Lane, Lynn Cadan, and Nancy Smith speak.

Shortly after Micki died and her body had been taken to the funeral home, I asked David to bring Joshua and Zoe to my house. When they arrived, we all sat in a circle, holding hands. I said to them, "Grandma's gone. She's not here anymore. I will need you all more than ever." No one spoke. They knew that, as close as we had been while Micki was dying, our little circle had drawn even closer together.

David, Josh, Zoe, and Katie were an important part of my support system. I was prepared for Micki's death. I had emerged from that long and painful period of my life with a part of my personality still intact. My close family had been with me constantly during that torturous time. Now I needed them to help me come out of that shell of sadness that had engulfed me for so many months. As it is said, Micki and I "had walked through the valley of the shadow of death." To some degree, we had taken that walk together. I had lost my wife, but emerged with my son, my grandchildren, and my close friends. I had emerged with a renewed appreciation for every living day.

That night, several hours after Micki had died, David asked me if I wanted to come to his house to sleep. I told him that I wanted to sleep at my house and didn't think that I needed any company. I needed to be alone that night. For the first time in nearly 40 years, I was truly physically alone.

Psychologically, I had been on a path to loneliness for several months. Now, I needed to experience the sense of isolation because I did not know, for the rest of my life, how long I would be alone.

At the funeral, the rabbi read my eulogy first. I had written about three characteristics that marked Micki's life: her great loyalty to her family and close friends, her wonderful intellectual curiosity, and her indomitable courage. I recalled that Micki had made some difficult choices during her lifetime; she didn't choose an easy path, and she faced death with strength and without compromise.

David was eloquent. He spoke about Micki's fine taste, her passion for living, and her devotion to her family. He was on the mark. As David noted, Micki believed she was living as long as she was open to learning something new. The intellectual challenge of pursuing her interest in archaeology continued almost to her death and sustained her. While she faced that challenge, despite the illness that ravaged her body, life went on. When she was too weak and tired to go any further, her life ended.

Sarah Lane also commented on Micki's intellectual fervor. She expressed awe at the way in which Micki took on the challenge of pursuing a master's degree at Yale at an age when most people were looking to slow down. Sarah said, "Micki fearlessly climbed mountains—mental, physical, and spiritual—in order to walk down the aisle, in the last stages of her life, to get her diploma."

Lynn Cadan was too overcome with emotion to speak. She had her husband, my longtime friend Alan, deliver her remarks. He spoke about Micki's attitude of tying up "loose ends" and living in the present as an attribute that Lynn remembered most. Because Micki did not want to dwell on her illness and eventual death, she made those long, last months easier and better for those around her. Lynn's description of Micki's determination was accurate. It was better for David. Better for Josh and Zoe. And better for me.

Nancy Smith was in Europe when Micki died. Micki had asked her to speak at her funeral. Although she could not get back to Connecticut in time, she gave me the remarks she had prepared. She wrote of Micki's sense of style, her determination, and the grace with which she faced her terminal illness. Nancy noted that the manner in which Micki faced the inevitable made it painful, but easier, for those surrounding Micki to accept it as well. Finally, she described Micki's love for David, Josh, Zoe, and me and the way in which Micki quietly, and with great dignity, prepared us for life without her. She never gave herself time to feel sorry for herself—she was more concerned with those who would follow after her.

There was a huge crowd at the funeral, which was held at our synagogue. Several people I had not seen in years came to the service. Friends flew in from Chicago and Virginia.

Micki had touched them all, and I was deeply grateful for their presence.

· · ·

In the Jewish tradition, which I observed, there are three periods of mourning. The first period of time begins after the burial and lasts for seven days. It is called *shiva*, which literally means "seven." Unlike a Catholic funeral, which usually follows a wake, both Jewish and Muslim tradition call for a burial as quickly as possible following death. During that time, the mourner does not do any work. The *shiva* period is one of acknowledgement that a death has occurred and that the person who has passed away will not come back. Friends and family visit the house and offer thoughts and condolences to the mourners. Since I follow a more liberal form of Judaism, I chose a period of *shiva* that lasted for three days and three nights. It ended with our family going to the synagogue for the Sabbath on Friday evening.

During that first mourning period, there was an overall air of sadness at our house. At the same time, I sensed a feeling of relief in my close friends, which I shared, knowing that Micki's suffering was over. Our house was filled with friends. We shared many stories, and everyone reached out to comfort David and me.

The second period of time in the Jewish tradition lasts

for 30 days. During that time, the mourner is expected to remain circumspect and refrain from any celebrations. In other words, socializing is limited. That period is called *shloshim.*

About two weeks after Micki died, I began to emerge socially, but with self-imposed limitations. Friends asked me to lunch or dinner, and I joined them. At most other times, I remained at home. It was a time for quiet reflection. David called me regularly, and I was with him and his family on weekends. I chose to observe that second period of mourning for two months.

I had a lot to remember about the last 39 years. I thought about how naïve Micki and I were to have married four months after we met. Our marriage had survived while many around us had fallen apart. I relived all the good things that had occurred during the gift of her nearly six years of remission. And, of course, I relived the terrible toll that cancer had taken on both of our lives. I had started missing Micki's companionship several months before she died, a loss that had come well before her death.

Despite the destruction that had been brought on by a terminal illness and eventual death, I recalled several things that had made the process more tolerable. I had a large circle of friends and a brother who had vast medical knowledge. I had a classmate who was a world-class oncologist. I had a wonderful and devoted son and grandchildren. I had the time to spend with my wife and did not need to worry about missing work. I had good insurance coverage and the resources to make sure that additional health care was available. For all those things, I was thankful. None of those factors could compensate for my loss, but they eased the pain.

My immediate family was the first pillar in my support system. I was fortunate to have a network of caring friends surrounding me. They were the second pillar in that system. Socialization with my friends became more frequent. In order to give my life some structure, I tried to schedule either lunch or dinner with one of my friends several times each week. They were all happy to oblige.

About two months after Micki's death, though I had good company, I felt my life was missing something else. For nearly 40 years, the first person I spoke with in the morning and the last person I spoke with at night had been a woman. I wanted to experience that kind of companionship again and decided to start dating. I chose a woman I had known casually for many years who had lost her husband five years earlier. As a widow, she was sensitive to my long passage over the last few years. Our first date went well.

The third pillar that lifted me up was my synagogue. We belonged to a small and intimate congregation where I knew many members. Although I am not religious, I also am not an atheist. Tradition and the teachings of my forefathers are important to me. Our congregation celebrates the Sabbath each Friday night with a service that is mostly music. For some time, I had been unable to attend services regularly because I had been caring for Micki. At each service, the entire congregation said a prayer for those who have passed away. Now, Friday night services became a ritual and a comfort. The congregants welcomed me, and I was part of something larger, both spiritually and literally.

Our congregation is led by a young rabbi. Michael is 37 years old but has the maturity of a sage. During Micki's last year, he called regularly and asked to visit. She usually refused his offer, because she associated Michael with religion, and because she was an atheist, God had no place in her life. She was also very private and preferred to concentrate on staying alive.

During the last few weeks of Micki's life, I accepted Michael's offer, and he visited me. Our conversations had nothing to do with religion and were a source of comfort. He was gentle and compassionate.

A few weeks before Micki died, David sat down with me. He was aware of my despair and my ever-narrowing outlook on life. He told me that, as difficult as the time was that I was going through, in the long run, it had to be "a period of personal growth" for me. My first reaction to that statement was that, at the age of 71, I did not need any more periods of personal growth.

I was wrong, and David was right. I saw this more clearly

in the first few weeks after Micki's death. During that entire downward spiral of her illness and death, I was becoming a changed person. I too had stared death in the face. I understood the meaning of living on borrowed time. I was made aware of the irreplaceable value of each living day. I shared the intimacy of a personal journey that can be experienced only by a partner with whom one has lived a loving life.

I began to realize that I had emerged from that period as a different person. I was certainly more aware of my mortality. I was also able to share a sense of empathy with those who were suffering. Losing my spouse had been a profound experience, and it allowed me to look deeply into my soul and come to grips with the kind of person that I was.

In the Jewish tradition, the third period of mourning lasts for 11 months from the date of burial. It is during this period that one experiences further acceptance of his or her loss and the realization occurs that it is time to "move on." In reality, that time varies, as each person is affected differently by the process of mourning.

Dr. Elisabeth Kübler-Ross, who wrote the classic *On Death and Dying,* was a pioneer in counseling for the personal trauma, grief, and grieving associated with death and dying. Many of her methods have been adopted by the modern hospice movement, and she developed the familiar model of five stages of grieving: denial, anger, bargaining, depression, and acceptance. Eventually, that model was applied to both the dying patient and to the surviving partner. If all the stages are experienced, some individuals may remain in one stage for a prolonged period of time. Micki began with denial, bargained for more time, and reached acceptance at the end of her ordeal. She spent very little time in between. She never exhibited anger. Her depression was real and hung over her condition for many years, though it could be alleviated, to some degree, by medication.

In retrospect, my grieving began more than a year before Micki's death, when I accepted that she was dying. The last two years of her life were a depressing process for me, and my depression continued for several weeks after her death. After Micki's passing, when I thought of what might have been, I could see that there had been a longer period of sadness that was not as destructive as deep depression. It was as if I were gradually emerging from being held under water. As time passed, I spent less time feeling submerged and more time floating on the waves. As time passed, the pendulum swung, and I spent more time having pleasant thoughts before reverting back to sadness for my loss.

When I was asked how I was feeling, weeks or months after Micki's death, I found a tendency for well-meaning friends to tell me I needed to allow more time to grieve. When I told people that I was doing well and moving on, it seemed as though some of them were disappointed by my response. This angered me greatly. I found it offensive for other people to tell me when and how I should grieve. Each survivor and each patient grieves differently.

For example, a friend of mine lost her husband to an unexpected heart attack. For her, the period of grieving began when she was told of her husband's death. For the spouse of a cancer patient, death is frequently a long and drawn-out process, and the grieving begins long before death occurs.

When I ran out of patience with those who tried to tell me about grieving, I replied, "Until you have walked in my shoes, you cannot tell me what I should go through in the grieving process."

It was my concept of marriage that guided me throughout Micki's illness. I took the words "in sickness and in health" to heart. I could not imagine that Micki's condition would have caused me to view our relationship more casually. At times, it became more intense, as her illness totally overwhelmed all aspects of our lives. It was not that my presence was needed medically. Rather, being together fulfilled an emotional need that we both seemed to share. Since Micki did not reach out to numerous friends, I was her obvious and desired companion. And I couldn't deny her that time.

In retrospect, objectively, that sense of complete devotion may not have been the best pattern for either of us. I cannot say with certainty that it is right for every spouse. The patient may not be served best by tying herself to very few people. Certainly, by finding some diversion, the surviving spouse may be able to lessen the incredible physical and emotional strain brought about by living with a terminal illness nearly every waking moment of every day. In the long run, that pattern is likely to have an adverse health effect on the surviving spouse. But for me, there was no other choice. It was the only way for me to live my life. That is who I am. I cannot judge others who find themselves in a similar situation. We must each find our own way.

For the last two years of Micki's life, I was overcome with helplessness. Shortly after her death, as I reflected on that time, I acknowledged that I had fulfilled several roles. In fact, while I felt hopeless, I was not. Micki was the patient, and she had one principal task. She needed to follow the doctor's directions. Then, as her condition deteriorated, she needed to concentrate on surviving and maintaining her quality of life. On the other hand, I had many roles. I was the primary caregiver. I maintained the household. I was available whenever my spouse needed me, and I became the spokesman for Micki, her doctors, and our family.

During my period of mourning, I finally realized that I had made a difficult situation better for Micki. That realization was part of my healing. Finally, I could look in the mirror and know that I had done everything that I could have done.

Many surviving spouses have said that they imagine that their spouse has not really died or will return. They are experiencing denial or engaging in "magical thinking." I did not have those thoughts. After I had accepted the inevitable and watched her deteriorate, it seemed as if Micki were dying in slow motion. To her, I am sure that each day passed too quickly. In either case, we had plenty of time to say good-bye. I had the opportunity to tell her, several times, how much she had meant to me. This opportunity to express my feelings before she died was a blessing, and this is a lesson I have shared with several of my friends: don't wait until it is too late.

There is a natural tendency to live in the past so a spouse can remain with us. In order to move on, you must be willing to relinquish the dead. You must be willing to let go. That is the only way to begin another life, to experience personal growth and to emerge from the depths of despair.

A few of my friends suggested that I compile a list of ways by which a spouse can survive the terrible ravages of a long terminal illness that may strike a loved one. There is no such list. There may be a few axioms: Be an active advocate for your spouse or partner, be at his or her side, and do your utmost to avoid depression. In truth, there is no one formula to provide guidance. In the end, everything else is personal. My strengths and weaknesses are different from those of others. Each of us will face adversity in our own way. We all make choices—and we live with those choices. It is not for me to judge the actions of others.

Self-pity is the worst enemy of the mourner. It can be destructive. It is a natural reaction to being left behind and confronted by silence, but it delays the healing process. Similarly, before and after death, depression can be overwhelming. It is not irrational, but it is as pervasive and as destructive as self-pity.

Moving on does not mean forgetting the person you have lost. You never do. Rather, it is choosing to live a life influenced by past experiences but shaped by the present and the future. Moving on may seem, at first, like a betrayal of your spouse. It is not. Your spouse is a memory, precious and wonderful, but no longer part of the present.

I know that every day is a gift, as life is a gift.

On a day like today, I am reminded of the emotional roller-coaster of the last several years. It has been several years since my wife, Micki, was first told that she had cancer. For me, the periods of sadness are fewer now, but they will never disappear. I have been scarred, but much has been gained by healing.

It is a beautiful day in an early spring. It is a season of rebirth. The trees are ready to blossom. Early flowers peep out of the ground. A new growth cycle has begun after a long New England winter.

Tonight, I will be celebrating a holiday. Seventeen friends will join me at my house along with my son and grandchildren. I have been preparing for this gathering for the last several days, and the time has been mixed with anticipation and sadness. This was a holiday that Micki threw herself into with passion and glee.

Around our table, we have all survived the winter. Only one person will be missing from our annual rite. Is it right to celebrate when the tears of loss are still with us? We celebrate because we must. We move on because those who are no longer with us would have wanted us to. There is really no alternative. It is not forsaking the past to move on; it is honoring the past and living in the present that guide me.

Edward H. Cantor
March 4, 2015

Appendix
Cancer Caregiver Resources

Books

Elisabeth Kübler-Ross, *On Death and Dying* (New York: Scribner, 1997)

Sherwin B. Nuland, MD, *How We Die: Reflections on Life's Final Chapter, New Edition* (New York: Vintage, 1995)

Siddhartha Mukherjee, *The Emperor of All Maladies: A Biography of Cancer* (New York: Scribner, 2011)

David Rieff, *Swimming in a Sea of Death: A Son's Memoir* (New York: Simon & Schuster, 2008)

Gail Sheehy, *Passages in Caregiving: Turning Chaos into Confidence* (New York: William Morrow, 2010)

Organizations

Caregiver Action Network, Washington, D.C.: www.caregiveraction.org

National Alliance for Caregiving, Bethesda, Maryland: www.caregiving.com

Today's Caregiver, National Center on Caregiving, San Francisco, California: www.caregiver.com

Well Spouse Foundation, Freehold, New Jersey: www.wellspouse.org

Acknowledgments

Many, many thanks go to Karen Siegel for her work as my editor. She is a talented professional and made several suggestions to improve my writing while remaining sensitive to the message I was trying to convey.

David Lesser was also kind enough to devote several hours to improving my work.

Most of Micki's close friends were described in the manuscript—Sarah Lane, Lynn Cadan and Nancy Smith—who were later joined by Eleanor Fulton, Kathy Teti, Marissa Ferguson, and Cindy Kramer.

It is always difficult to list those friends who provided me with much-needed support, because they were many and I run the risk of omitting some names. With that reservation and apology in advance, I cannot say enough about the support given to me by Alan Cadan, Frosty Smith, Les Seligson, Dick Ferguson, Tom Corradino, and David Lesser. I was continually encouraged by messages or visits from my Yale classmates Joe Schwartz, Vince Teti, Sherwin Goldman, Andy Block, and Jamie McLane. They were later joined by my Yale roommates Dave Ryan and Jim Hanson. My law school roommate, Bill Carmell, was in constant touch, and Ivar Mitchell tried his best to keep me laughing. Alan Lovins and Steve Floman provided needed friendship and counseling. Rochelle Kanell, Doug Fitzsimmons, Hanon Russell, and Mike Hoben lent a sympathetic ear, and Rise Siegel led me out of darkness. To all my friends, named and not named: I could not have emerged intact without your help, and I am forever grateful.